# The Patient's Guide to Hair Restoration

WILLIAM R. RASSMAN, M.D.
ROBERT M. BERNSTEIN, M.D.

Contributions by
Robert McClellan, M.D., Roy Jones, M.D.
Marc Pomerantz, M.D., and Richard C. Shiell. M.D.

*The authors wish to acknowledge and thank Heather Kubinec, Megan Schulte, and Margaret O'Brien for their invaluable input and efforts in editing this manuscript.*

Published by New Hair Institute, Inc.
9911 West Pico Boulevard, Suite 301, Los Angeles, CA 90035
International Standard Book Number: 0-9701405-1-7

# TABLE OF CONTENTS

# INTRODUCTION

The goal of the Patient's Guide to Hair Transplantation is to provide you with the tools to make the best possible choices in dealing with your hair loss. The sixth edition includes revisions, updates, new photos and two entirely new chapters on Follicular Unit Transplantation and repairs.

Choosing to have hair restoration surgery is an important decision. You are seeking a treatment that will permanently alter your appearance. In today's procedure-dominated medical industry, many doctors make decisions based upon their own economic interests rather than considering what is in the best interest of their patients. Therefore, it is crucial that you take the time to educate yourself about both the hair transplant procedure and the physician who will perform your surgery. This will help to ensure that you have a safe procedure and that you achieve the best possible cosmetic result.

Cost is one consideration in choosing who will perform your surgery; having a state-of the-art procedure, performed by the most qualified and experienced physician, is far more important. Physician ignorance regarding the most up-to-date therapies is far more common than many people realize; this is true even for those doctors who perform hair transplantation with great frequency. During our many years in practice, we have seen patients confused by doctors who fail to carefully evaluate their patients and who offer only vague treatment plans. It is common for the patient who has made poor decisions to be ill informed, or not informed at all.

Although the general state of surgical hair restoration has improved significantly over the past six years, since NHI first published Follicular Transplantation in 1995, this "gold standard" is still elusive to most physicians. To be performed properly, Follicular Unit Transplantation requires a surgeon who understands both the artistic and technical complexities of transplanting large numbers of very small grafts, a surgical team specifically trained in stereo-microscopic dissection, and facilities that are specifically equipped to perform this labor intensive, exacting procedure.

Many physicians do not take the time to explain to patients the details of sophisticated medical technologies if they don't offer these services in their own practices. Unfortunately, physician adaptation to the newer, more revolutionary techniques has been surprisingly slow. Even new breakthrough medications, such as Propecia, are often not discussed by hair transplant surgeons.

Becoming an educated consumer is critical for those who are interested in getting the best possible results. Follicular Unit Transplantation techniques can now produce hair transplants that are indistinguishable from your normal hair, but to get these results, the surgeon and his team must be expert in performing this procedure. Take plenty of time in your research and, of equal importance, be conscientious in choosing your physician. This book intends to provide you with the tools needed to make an intelligent and informed decision; one that is right for you.

# 1

# A BRIEF HISTORY OF HAIR

Throughout history, hair has been an important symbol. The significance of hair as an indicator of gender, and social, religious and professional status has been as great as that of clothing, jewelry, tattoos, weapons, and even crowns. The importance of hair goes back at least as far as the Neolithic Age. Several years ago, a man's body was found frozen in a glacier near the Austrian-Italian border. Because he looked like modern man, it was first thought that he had died only a few years before. Upon examination of his clothing and weapons, archaeologists concluded that he had been frozen for more than 5,000 years. It is likely that this preserved Neolithic man wore his hair in the fashionable cut and style of that age. His hair was neatly cut to a length of 3.5 inches, and his beard was trimmed.

In Ancient Egypt, sons of the Pharaoh wore their hair tied in a distinctive bun on the right side of the head just behind the ear. The Pharaoh himself was never seen without a wig. Even today, male and female English judges wear obviously artificial horsehair wigs when they preside in court.

The oldest known medical text is an Egyptian papyrus scroll. Its remedies include an ointment for restoring lost hair, consisting of equal parts crocodile fat and hippopotamus dung. The physician who wrote the text recommended that one rub this concoction into the bald scalp.

The ancient Greek physician, Hippocrates, recognized a connection between the sexual organs and baldness. He may have been the first to record the observation that eunuchs (men castrated before puberty) did not become bald.

Hippocrates' own baldness stimulated his interest in the subject of hair loss. His prescription for preventing hair loss was the application of a mixture of cumin, pigeon droppings, horseradish, and nettles to the scalp. In fact, the area of permanent hair that encircles the back and sides of the head is sometimes referred to as the Hippocratic wreath.

Dating back to Biblical times, the tale of Samson is one of the familiar examples of man's concern over hair loss. Samson had the strength to destroy the Philistines as long as his hair remained long and uncut. As soon as Delilah cut his hair, he lost all of his strength.

Early Christian monks and priests shaved the hair on the crown of the head to create a tonsure. This highly visible mark proclaimed their vow of chastity to the world. It symbolized their lack of concern with worldly vanities and riches; it also expressed their personal dedication to God. During the Middle Ages, Christian society saw an emphasis of concern with the spiritual side of life and a studied neglect of physical functions. The tonsure became so extreme that, upon taking orders, a monk shaved his head almost completely bare, so that only a narrow fringe of hair remained encircling his head.

During the time of King Louis XIV of France, elaborate wigs became fashionable for the aristocracy. Some of these wigs incorporated paraphernalia such as model ships and cages with live birds. The more complex constructions often weighed 15-20 pounds. Known for luxuriant hair in his youth, King Louis began this practice and may have adopted the fashion to disguise his balding as he grew older. Elaborate wigs continued to be a class status and fashion symbol until the middle of the eighteenth century.

Hair has also been an important symbol of rank and religion in Asia. Buddhist monks shaved their heads completely. Japanese Samurai warriors shaved the front and top of the head and drew the long back and side hair into a complex top-knot. Even modern day Sumo wrestlers wear their hair in a distinctive knot at the back although they do not shave the front and top. The ubiquitous queue or pigtail of Chinese men, a long single braid worn down the back, was a symbol of their bondage to a lord, landowner, or to the Emperor. Most urban Chinese men cut off their queues after the revolution in 1920, but the custom persisted in many rural areas. During the revolution, any man found wearing a queue was publicly humiliated; his hair was cut off and burned.

Today, hair continues to be an important part of self-expression, and can function as a symbol of attitude, culture, and religion. Hair, or the lack of it, is of great significance to rock singers, punks, Rastafarians, Hare Krishnas, Orthodox Jews, Sikhs, Sufis, Buddhists and Hindus. Hair is important to our self-image and self-identity, and for both men and women, it is a universal symbol of youth.

# 2

# HAIR AND ITS FUNCTIONS

*During Napoleon's retreat from Russia after the defeat of 1812, more that 450,000 of the original force of 500,000 died of all causes: battle wounds, heat, starvation, and especially the cold. Many of them went to sleep, and froze to death. Baron Larrey, the army's Chief Surgeon, noticed that bald men died of the cold before those with hair.*
*- Nigel Nicholson*

The condition of one's hair is an important indicator of age and the body's general state of health. Other similar indicators, such as skin condition, muscular coordination, brightness of the eye and alertness of manner, are often more subtle or may be masked by clothing. Hair, however, is usually in plain sight. There are associations and social reactions that may result if one's hair is gray or a man is bald. It has been thought that such reactions are were based on primal judgments, such as whether the person is fit for warfare, reproduction, and or active labor. A full, glossy head of hair is a clear signal that one is youthful, vigorous, and therefore, desirable.

Hair is composed of a complex protein called keratin. Of the human body's three basic compounds: , proteins, fats, and carbohydrates; the synthesis of protein requires the greatest investment of energy. When a person becomes ill or malnourished, his/her hair stops growing. When illness or malnutrition is severe or prolonged, the hair may fall out (the medical term for this is telogen effluvium). The resumption of hair growth is a sign that recovery has begun. Science continues to explore why hair grows or fails to grow, and why it falls out in some people, but not in others.

Mammals share several characteristics. Most mammals bear live offspring (as opposed to laying eggs) and nurture their young with milk made in special glands on the female's body. Mammals are warm-blooded, that is, they maintain constant body temperature independent of the outside temperature. Hair is a feature shared by all mammals; and like many mammals, man's skin is covered with hair. Human skin has more hair follicles per unit of surface area than the skin of most other primates; which this is surprising, since as most primates appear to be so much hairier than humans. This impression is caused by the greater length and coarseness of the individual hair shafts in primates such as monkeys and apes. In contrast, the majority of human body hair consists of a very fine, almost invisible, type of hair called vellus hair.

Human hair is classified into two main types: fine, vellus hair; and the coarser, more visible terminal hair. Except for the palms of the hands and the soles of the feet, most of the human body's areas of seemingly bare skin are actually covered with very fine vellus hairs that may be almost invisible except to under very close or microscopic inspection. There are several distinct subtypes of terminal hair. For example, eyelash hairs, called cilia, are different from head and body hair. Pubic (groin) and axillary (armpit) hairs are also different from terminal hairs on the head and are associated with different types of glands in the skin. Even scalp hairs have several different sub-groupings. For example, there is a fringe of very fine hair surrounding the circumference of the head. This hair gives a transitional gradation of thickness from the bare skin appearance of the vellus hair to the dense, thick hair of the crown. Similarly, the hair above the ears or at the base of the neck is not as coarse as that of the crown.

The reasons we have hair and the functions of its growth patterns are not completely understood. Our pre-historic ancestors were much hairier than we are today; the reason for the decreased hairiness of modern man is unknown, although it is reasonable to assume that it parallel the use of clothing for warmth and protection. Hair serves as insulation from the cold; however, this does not explain why different human groups have distinct patterns of hair growth. Most people of Asian descent have very sparse body and facial hair, but some of these peoples such as the Inuit, Tibetans and Mongols people, inhabit some of the coldest regions on earth. Hair has the additional function of extending the sensory capability of the skin beyond its surface. Although human hair lacks the wealth of sensory nerve fibers found at the root of whiskers of some animals, each hair has a nerve fiber going to the bulb of the hair follicle. Mechanical displacement of each hair causes a sensation, an awareness of movement. For example, when an ant or fly walks on one's arm, one feels the displacement of hairs caused by the insect.

Hair plays a role in the defense mechanisms of most fur-bearing animals as well. When an animal confronts a potential enemy, its fur bristles, standing on end to make the animal appear to be larger and more threatening. In dogs, this response is most visible in the neck area where the neck hairs, called hackles, rise. In cats, the most visible response may be in the tail. An extreme example of the use of hair for self-defense occurs in porcupines: their quills, which are modified hairs, stand out from the body when the animal feels threatened. Porcupines have converted a reflex, that in most animals is purely defensive, into a formidable weapon. In modern man, with relatively sparse body hair, only vestigial traces of these reactions remain. A separate, tiny muscle connects the lower portion of each hair shaft with the underside of the skin. When you are frightened, cold or angry, these small muscles, called erector pili muscles, contract, causing your hair to stand on end.

Each hair shaft also contains a small gland called the sebaceous gland, located next to the hair shaft. Sebaceous glands make a yellow, fatty substance called sebum that lubricates the hair. Each time the erector pili muscle contracts, the gland is squeezed, and a small amount of lubricant is applied to the surface of the hair. Hair, along with skin pigmentation, is the major natural protection that we have against the sun's harmful ultra-violet rays. Scalp hair also plays an important role in preventing mechanical trauma to the skull. Hair acts as a "dry lubricant" in areas that rub, such as under the arms and in the groin, and serves to disperse pheromones (body secretions that are involved in sexual attraction).

Hair is integral to our body image and can have a profound influence on our self-esteem and self-confidence. There is no other part of the human anatomy that can be changed or manipulated so easily. Hair can be groomed, styled, waved, straightened, dyed, braided, or cut, and, unlike tattoos or body piercing, changes made to our hair can be completely reversed. Hair serves as a means of self-expression, and the loss of this form of self-expression in people who are going bald may account, at least in part, for the despair that they may experience. For all of its simple appearance, hair is a complex and valuable organ. Although we usually think of hair only in terms of the visible portion of the hair shafts, each hair, along with its muscle and sebaceous gland, must be working properly to maintain a healthy head of hair.

## Anatomy & Physiology of Hair

Anatomically, hair is a part of the skin. As hair is physically distinct however, it is among the structures known as skin appendages. Other skin appendages include sweat glands, fingernails and toenails. Skin is composed of three main layers. The outer layer of skin is the epidermis. This layer is less than a millimeter in thickness and is composed of dead cells that are in a constant state of sloughing and replacement. As dead cells are lost, new ones from the growing layer below replace them. Beneath the epidermis is the dermis, a tough layer of connective tissue that is about 2 to 3 mm thick on the scalp. This layer gives the skin its strength, and contains both sebaceous glands and sweat glands. Beneath the dermis is a layer of subcutaneous fat and connective tissue.

The larger sensory nerve branches and the blood vessels that nourish the skin run deep into this layer. In the scalp, the lower portions of the hair follicles (the bulbs) are found in the upper part of this fatty layer. The hair follicle measures about 3-4 mm in length and produces one to four hair shafts, each about 0.1 mm in width. It is a complex structure comprised of three main layers. The outer layer, called the outer root sheath or trichelemma, surrounds the follicle in the dermis and then blends into the epidermis on the surface of the skin, forming the structure commonly referred to as the pore (from which the hair emerges).

The middle layer, the inner root sheath, is composed of three parts (Huxley layer, Henly layer, and cuticle), with the cuticle being the innermost portion that touches the hair shaft. Interestingly, the cuticle is formed by a layer of overlapping cells that interlock with the cuticle of the hair shafts shaft (matrix cells). This mechanism holds the hair shaft securely in place, but also allows it to grow in length.

The hair shaft itself is also composed of three layers. The cuticle, the outer layer just described, forms the surface of the hair and is what we see as the hair shaft emerges from the follicle. The middle layer, the cortex comprises the bulk of the hair shaft and is what gives hair its strength. It is composed of an organic protein called keratin, the same material that comprises rhinoceros horn and deer antlers. The center, or core, of the hair shaft, is the medulla, and is only present in terminal hair follicles. The lower portion of each hair follicle widens into a region called the bulb, which contains the matrix cells. The size of the bulb and the number of matrix cells will determine the width of the fully-grown hair.

Below each follicle is a small, collection of specialized cells, called the dermal papillae. The dermal papillae fit into a hollow in the widened base of the hair shaft. For many years, scientists thought that hair growth originated from the dermal papillae. Recent evidence has shown that the growth center extends from the dermal papillae all the way up to the region of the follicle where the sebaceous glands are attached. It is now believed that the primary function of the dermal papillae is to regulate follicular growth and differentiation. If the dermal papillae are removed (this sometimes happens during a hair transplant), the hair follicle is able to regenerate a new one, although the growth of the new hair will be delayed.

The normal human scalp contains about 100,000-150,000 follicles that produce thick terminal hair. For comparison, the human body has approximately 5 million follicles that produce the fine, vellus hair. At any given time, about 90% of terminal hairs on one's head are actively growing. This phase, called anagen, can last from 2-7 years, though the average is about three. Scalp hair grows at a rate of about 0.44 mm/day (or 1/2 inch per month). The other remaining 10% of scalp hairs are in a resting state called telogen that, in a normal scalp, lasts about three months. When a hair enters its resting phase, growth stops, the bulb detaches from the papilla, and the shaft is either pulled out (as when combing one's hair) or pushed out when the new shaft starts to grow. When a hair is pulled out, or falls out on its own, a small, white swelling is found at the bottom of the hair shaft. Most people assume that this is the growth center of the hair, but it is just the clubbed, detached lower end of the hair shaft. The dermal papillae remain in the scalp.

Humans lose about 100 hairs per day; everyone has a few hairs stuck to the comb each time they comb their hair. The presence of a large number of hairs on the comb, in the sink, or in the tub can be the first sign of excessive hair loss. One of the most interesting things about hair is that, in contrast to the commonly held notion that it grows as individual strands, it actually emerges from the scalp in groups of one to four (and sometimes even five or six). The reason for this is that hair follicles are not solitary structures, but are arranged in the skin in naturally occurring groups called follicular units. Although skin pathologists recognized this fact in the early 1980's, its profound importance in hair transplantation surgery was not appreciated until the mid-1990's. The use of naturally occurring, individual follicular units has revolutionized modern hair transplantation.

away.

## Hormones

Hormones are biochemical substances produced by various glands throughout the body. These glands secrete their products directly into the bloodstream in order to spread them throughout the body. These chemicals are very powerful and minute amounts of them have profound effects upon the body.

The primary male sex hormone is testosterone. Testosterone and other related hormones that have masculinizing effects are produced primarily in the testicles. This means that the hormonal levels that are seen in adults do not reached significant levels until the testicles develop and enlarge during puberty. These same hormones are the cause of many changes that occur in puberty: deepening of the voice, growth of facial hair, development of body odor, change in the muscular development, and change in body shape. These hormones that cause acne and beard growth can also signal the beginning of baldness. The presence of androgens, testosterone, and its related hormone DHT, cause some follicles to regress and die. In addition to the testicles, the adrenal glands located above each of our kidneys, produce androgenic hormones; this is true for both sexes. In females, ovaries, like testicles, are a source of hormones that can affect hair.

The relationship between a man's testicles and hair loss has been recognized for centuries. In societies that had harems, guards were castrated to prevent sexual activity between the guards and women of the harem. In all of those societies, it was observed that men who were castrated before puberty did not become bald. Early in the 20th century, castration was common among patients with certain types of mental illness. Castration seemed to have a calming effect, and noticeably reduced sex drive in patients. A psychiatrist discovered the specific relationship between testosterone and hormonally induced hair loss during this time. The doctor noted that the identical twin brother of one patient was profoundly bald while the mentally ill twin had a full head of hair. The doctor decided to determine the effect of treating his patient with testosterone, which had recently become available as a drug. He injected his patient, the hairy twin, with testosterone to see what would happen. Within weeks, the hairy twin began to lose all but his wreath of permanent hair, just like his normal twin. The doctor stopped administrating testosterone; however, his patient never regained his full head of hair.

The hormone believed to be most directly involved in androgenetic alopecia is dihydrotestosterone (DHT). DHT is formed by the action of the enzyme 5-a reductase on testosterone. DHT acts by binding to special receptor sites on the cells of hair follicles to cause the specific changes associated with balding. Among other effects, DHT decreases the length of the anagen (growing) cycle, and increases the telogen (resting) phase, so that with each new cycle the hair shaft becomes progressively smaller.

In men, 5-a reductase activity is higher in the balding area. Women have half the amount of 5-a reductase overall as compared to men, but have higher levels of the enzyme aromatase, especially in their frontal hairlines. Aromatase decreases the formation of DHT, and its presence in women may help to explain why female hair loss is somewhat different than hair loss in males.

## Time

The mere presence of the necessary genes and hormones is insufficient to cause baldness. Hair loss also requires exposure of susceptible hair follicles to the responsible hormones. The time required for hair loss to start due to hormone exposure  varies from one individual to another, and relates to a person's genetic expression and to the levels of testosterone and DHT in his bloodstream. Significantly, hair loss does not occur all at once, but is cyclical. People who are losing their hair experience alternating periods of slow hair loss, rapid hair loss, and even stability (no increase in hair loss). The factors that cause the rate of loss to speed up or slow down are unknown.

## Stress

When the body experiences stress caused by a traumatic experience, nutritional deficiency, or illness, the rate of hair loss can increase. An example of this occurred in a man whose four-year-old child died. Within just a few months, he lost all but the permanent wreath of hair around his head.

Women's hair seems to be more sensitive to the effects of stress than men's hair. This may be because women with a genetic predisposition towards hair loss usually have a higher percentage of fragile miniaturized hair. It is important to note that stress generally causes the type of hair loss referred to as telogen effluvium. This is very different from androgenetic alopecia. Telogen effluvium is the reversible shedding of hair in the resting phase when the body senses that it needs to divert its energies elsewhere. Therefore, stress temporarily changes the amount of hair that is shed, but the lost hair is likely to grow back.

## Fiction
## Lack of Blood Supply

Some assert that a lack of blood supply contributes to hair loss. Bald skin gradually loses some of its blood supply and, consequently, it becomes thin and shiny. These changes, however, are secondary to the loss of hair. Hair follicles are one of the most rapidly metabolizing tissues in the body; their high metabolic rate demands an excellent blood supply to carry oxygen and other nutrients to the cells. If the blood supply diminishes, the follicle cells    wither and die. Growing hair requires the proper nutrition that comes with a good blood supply. When hair follicles are transplanted into skin grafts or scar tissue, both of which have a relatively poor blood supply, the presence of the grafted hair causes the local blood supply to increase.

## Clogged Pores

This claim usually accompanies microscopic photographs of an empty follicle clogged with a heaped up waxy substance that prevented the hair from growing.    There is no scientific evidence that clogged pores could interfere with hair growth. Common sense is sufficient to refute these claims. Why would pores be clogged on the top of the scalp and not on the back and sides?  In addition, everyone has had an ingrown hair at one time or another. An ingrown hair occurs when a hair grows through intact skin where there is no opening. If a hair can force its way through skin, it can certainly grow through soft, waxy sebum at the bottom of an empty follicle.  It is also important to note that the lubricants that normally coat the surface of the hair shaft are produced even when a hair shaft falls out. Since there is no hair shaft surface for these lubricants to coat, they pile up in the bottom of the follicle space. If clogged pores caused baldness, women would be as bald as men.

## Lack of Air Circulation to the Head

Folklore says that men who constantly wear hats are more likely to become bald, as hats prevent air from circulating to the head. Hair follicles get their oxygen through the bloodstream, however, rather than from ambient air.  Factors that affect only the exposed part of the hair do not injure the growing portion of the hair root.  One exception to this is that constant traction on the hair follicles, such as from the continuous wearing of "corn rows" or very tight braids, can cause permanent hair loss. This condition is called traction alopecia, and is distinct from androgenetic alopecia.

## Preventing Hair Loss

Many over-the-counter lotions and drugs claim to restore lost hair. Whether sold through drug stores, salons or mass media, most are useless. A 1989 Supreme Court decision prevents these potions from being advertised or sold in the United States as medications that prevent hair loss or promote the regrowth of lost hair; however, such claims are still made.

Charlatans of every age have eagerly seized upon each new scientific wonder to profit from a gullible public. Excepting cancer and arthritis, hair restoration has been one of the most fertile areas for medical nostrums. For example, in the same year that the principle of the magnetic field was described, "magnetic" and "electric" hairbrushes for the prevention and treatment of baldness appeared on the market. Concoctions that claimed to be "snake oils" were also sold for the treatment of arthritis and baldness. In hindsight, it is understandable that an unsophisticated person, who was crippled by pain from arthritis and who lived at a time when there was no better treatment for his illness, might be desperate enough to try "snake oil" as a treatment for arthritis. However, until the Supreme Court decision banning their promotion, ads for products that claimed to be able to restore hair filled the television airwaves. Infomercials complete with real doctors, pictures, and testimonials promoted these worthless potions every day. Even today, it is difficult for the layperson to differentiate between fact and fiction when it comes to hair loss remedies. There are two FDA approved medications to treat androgenetic alopecia. Though they have limited benefit, they may be useful for many. These two medications, minoxidil and finasteride, are discussed in detail in the chapter titled "Drugs to Prevent Hair Loss."

# 4

## How Bald Will I Be?

For most men, the first sign of excessive hair loss is the appearance of more hairs than usual on their comb or brush. Some men first notice excess hair at the bottom of the bathtub or on their fingers after shampooing. Men who are going to lose a very large amount of hair usually see the first signs between the ages of 17 and 25. Men whose fathers or grandfathers on either side of the family were bald, will probably notice the hair loss before someone who has no apparent family history of baldness. Sensitized to the possibility of hair loss, they are waiting for the process to begin.

As soon as he notices any sign of excess hair loss, the typical man will rush to a mirror to do a hair-by-hair inspection of his frontal hairline. If he cannot see any sign of hair loss, he may compare his present hairline with one from a recent photo. He will continue to closely observe his hairline every day. He will also attempt to keep, a hair-by-hair count of the hair on his comb, his fingers, or in the tub. Dark-haired men notice the hair loss process earlier that light-haired men do.

Some men resort to potions, regimens, or shampoos. A good shampoo will clean your hair, but no shampoo will stop the balding process. These approaches may offer the comfort of doing something during the early phase of hair loss, but eventually the futility of these measures will become obvious. What can a man do? How can he cope with the disintegration of his youthful looks? What will he look like without hair? How will this affect his ability to attract a partner? How will his professional life be affected? Will the change affect his ability to gain a promotion? Will his ability to sell his product line to clients be affected? Anything that erodes self-confidence can have a negative effect upon all aspects of life.

The first step is to make an assessment of the extent of hair loss. One way to do this is to compare your present hairline with your hairline in a recent photograph. This will give you an approximation of the amount and rate of your hair loss. An unknown factor for most men is the extent of hair loss in the crown area. Looking in a mirror is one way to appraise the loss at the back of your head. The best way to accurately assess the hair loss in this area is to have a photo taken of the back of your head. For an accurate reading, the picture must be taken with a flash. Almost every man who has significant loss in this area is surprised by the results. Another way is to ask your significant other, barber or hairdresser.

If hair loss is bothering you, a visit to a physician who specializes in hair restoration is a worthwhile step. A thorough medical history and examination of the scalp can reveal the extent and trends of your hair loss. With the use of special magnifying apparatuses, a physician can specifically measure the degree of hair loss in various areas of the scalp. This establishes a baseline from which your hair loss can be graded over time. If you decide to treat your hair loss with minoxidil or finasteride, a repeat examination in 6-12 months may show the effectiveness of the treatment. Careful assessment of hair loss is critical to accurate prediction of the rate and extent of future hair loss.

Once you have confirmed your hair loss, you should compare your degree of baldness with the standard charts that follow. These charts have been adapted from the patterns described by Dr. O'Tar Norwood. They depict the most common configurations of male pattern baldness. There are seven grades of hair loss in the main series and five grades of a variation called the A series. Comparing the front and back of your scalp with these diagrams can tell you where you stand now. Discussion with a knowledgeable physician can give you an idea of future hair loss.

The next step is to decide whether to accept your hair loss or take measures to stop or reverse the process.   If you are less than 45 years old, you might consider using minoxidil or seeing a doctor for a prescription for finasteride. One option is to obtain a hairpiece. Another option is to replace lost hair with your own natural, permanent hair via hair transplant surgery.

# Norwood Classifications
## Male Pattern Baldness • Main Classes

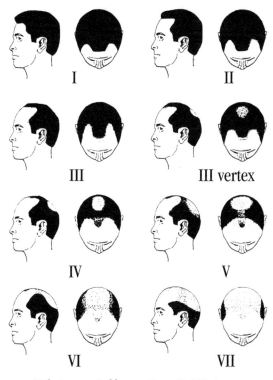

I

II

III

III vertex

IV

V

VI

VII

## Male Pattern Baldness • Type "A" Variants

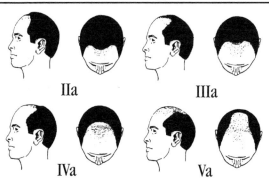

IIa

IIIa

IVa

Va

# 5

## DRUGS TO PREVENT HAIR LOSS

For years, worthless hair potions have been sold to men to rub on their balding scalps. Finally, two effective medications exist for the treatment of hair loss.

### Minoxidil (Rogaine)

Minoxidil, as an oral medication, has been available for a number of years for the treatment of high blood pressure. Because of its serious side effects on the heart and general circulation, it is only used with patients unsuccessfully treated with the maximum doses of other drugs. During its use as a treatment for high blood pressure, it was observed that some patients who were taking minoxidil began growing hair in unusual areas of the body, such as the forehead and on the backs of their hands. It was thought that applying minoxidil directly to a bald scalp might cause hair growth in that area. If hair growth occurred without other side effects, then it might be useful to healthy balding men. It was then proven that when a topical solution of minoxidil was applied to bald scalps, some men grew hair in the areas where it was applied.

Rogaine, manufactured by Pharmacia & Upjohn Inc., is the brand name for the topically applied minoxidil solution. It can be purchased without a prescription in either 2% or 4% concentrations. Although the mechanism that causes minoxidil to stimulate hair growth is not known, it probably works by prolonging the hair follicle growth cycle. Controlled studies on minoxidil show that it only grows hair in the vertex (back part) of a man's scalp, and only in areas that are not completely bald. It does not usually re-grow hair in the front part of a bald scalp.

It appears that minoxidil's effects may only be temporary. Since testosterone is always present in the blood stream, this hormone eventually overcomes the effects of the minoxidil so that over time, men using minoxidil continue to bald, although at a somewhat slower rate. The concomitant use of minoxidil and finasteride (see next section) may circumvent this problem, as there is evidence that in some cases these drugs may act synergistically.

Before trying minoxidil, be aware that it may take 6-12 months before results start to appear. In addition, unless the medication is used consistently twice a day, it will not be effective. For most men, minoxidil does not grow any significant amount of new hair. The primary action of minoxidil is to thicken already existing hair that has thinned or miniaturized, and most patients who do grow hair, grow only short, thin fuzz.

The majority of patients who experience benefits from minoxidil see only a delay or decrease in hair loss. For many men, the effects are first noticed when they stop using the medication. Once the drug use is stopped, the previous pattern of hair loss resumes, and any positive effects are lost within two to three months, even if the medication had been used for many years. This same limitation applies to other drugs used for hair loss.

Many patients are attracted to minoxidil because of its seeming lower cost compared to other methods of hair replacement. However, because the effects of minoxidil are temporary, the lifetime cost of using minoxidil can be more expensive than the cost of hairpieces or surgical treatments for hair loss.

Minoxidil is often prescribed in conjunction with other medications such as topical retinoic acid (Retin-A) to increase its topical penetration. These medications can greatly increase the systemic absorption of minoxidil and may increase the risk of potential side effects, including severe scalp irritation. The prescribing information provided by Upjohn specifically states Rogaine should not be used with other topical agents including topical corticosteroids, retinoids, petrolatum and/or other agents that are known to enhance drug absorption. One should not use Rogaine if one's scalp is sunburned or becomes irritated.

A problem unique to patients using the combined mixture of minoxidil/Retin-A occurs when scalp irritation begins and the patient is afraid to stop the Retin-A since this would also mean discontinuation of the minoxidil (and the likely outcome of subsequent hair loss). These patients often continue the mixture in spite of the development of severe scalp irritation. This can result in infection, scarring and permanent hair loss.

The early studies with minoxidil were on balding men, but it appears that minoxidil may actually be more effective for women experiencing hair loss. This is probably because women usually exhibit diffuse hair loss. Minoxidil, then, would not be applied to bald areas, but in areas of thinning. Some doctors recommend minoxidil before and after hair transplantation to decrease or prevent the temporary loss of hair that sometimes occurs with newly placed grafts, however, this use has not yet been proven to be reliably effective.

Finally, although it seems that the topical preparation of minoxidil is innocuous, the long-term safety unknown. As with many medications, the clinical trials with minoxidil occurred over a very limited period of time. Since the medication must be continued for years, we may presently be unaware of potential long-term problems.

## Finasteride (Propecia)

Propecia is an oral medication, manufactured by Merck, that blocks the conversion of testosterone to dihydrotestosterone (DHT), the hormone largely responsible for male pattern baldness. It does this by inhibiting the action of the type II 5-alpha reductase enzyme that is present in higher concentrations in and around the hair follicles of balding men with androgenetic alopecia.

Finasteride causes significant drops in both scalp and blood levels of DHT. Its effectiveness is believed to be related to both of these factors. In patients taking finasteride 1-mg/day, serum DHT levels decreased by 68.4%. Serum testosterone levels actually increased by 9.1% but remained within the normal range.

Finasteride was originally marketed for use in prostate enlargement in men over 50 (the prostate also has the type II enzyme). This medication, in a 5-mg per day dose, is sold under the name Proscar. In the treatment of prostate problems, finasteride 5-mg has produced breast tenderness and breast enlargement. It has also caused impotence and decreased sexual interest in a small number of men.

In January 1998, the FDA approved finasteride 1-mg/day (Propecia) for the treatment of male pattern baldness. The phase III human trials, using the 1-mg dose, involved 1,553 men, ages 18 to 41, with Class II Vertex, III Vertex, IV or V balding patterns, i.e. men with mild to moderate hair loss. After two years, results showed that 83% of the men taking finasteride either kept their hair or grew more, while only 17% continued to lose hair. In the crown, 30% showed slight improvement, 31% showed moderate improvement and 5% showed great improvement. In the front, 38% showed slight improvement, 4% showed moderate improvement, and none great improvement.

Hair counts showed an average gain of 86 hairs in a one-inch circle at the end of one year. These hairs were significantly larger than the fine, miniaturized hair seen in balding, but they did not necessarily assume the full weight and diameter of the patient's original hair.

## Sexual Dysfunction

Although uncommon, there can be side effects from finasteride at the 1-mg dose. At least one study has shown that these side effects include decreased libido (1.8%), impotence (1.3%), and decreased volume of ejaculate (1.2%). It is important to note that there was a small incidence of these problems in the control group as well. Altogether, 3.8% of men taking finasteride 1-mg experienced some form of sexual dysfunction versus 2.1% in men treated with a placebo.

Most reported cases of sexual dysfunction occurred soon after starting the medication, but there have been reports of sexual dysfunction that have occurred at later points in time. The sexual side effects were reversed in all men who discontinued therapy, and in 58% of those who continued treatment. When the medication was stopped, side effects generally went away within weeks, but occasionally took longer.

If sexual side effects occur, they generally begin well before finasteride has had a chance to visibly effect hair growth. Therefore, men who experience side effects can discontinue the Propecia at this time without losing any additional hair. Like minoxidil, when finasteride is discontinued, one loses the hair gained or preserved by the medication, not more. In effect, the patient returns to the level of balding that would have been had he never used the drugs in the first place.

## Gynecomastia

Adverse reactions related to the breast, including breast tenderness or enlargement (gynecomastia), occurred in 0.4% of men taking finasteride 1-mg (Propecia), but this was no greater than in the control group. Breast enlargement in patients taking finasteride may be due to its ability to block the conversion of testosterone to DHT. This, in turn, may cause more testosterone to be converted to estrogen, with estrogen then stimulating breast tissue. There have been a few cases of breast cancer in patients on the 5-mg dose, but a causative relationship with finasteride has not been established.

## Effects on PSA

Finasteride causes an approximate 1/3 decrease in serum PSA (prostate specific antigen) in normal men. It may also blunt the rise of PSA levels in patients with prostate enlargement and in patients who have developed prostate cancer. Since PSA is used to screen for prostate cancer, there is concern that the use of Propecia may interfere with the detection of this disease. It is important that you make your personal physician aware that you are taking finasteride so that he or she can take into account any effects that finasteride may have on your PSA.

There has been one small study that suggested that finasteride at 5-mg may increase the risk of prostatic carcinoma in older patients who have an already significantly elevated PSA. However, the methodology of this study has been seriously questioned and data from other studies do not support its conclusion.

## Teratogenecity in Women

Finasteride should not be taken by women of childbearing age as birth defects in male offspring can occur if significant amounts of the drug are absorbed during fetal development. Pregnant women are warned not to handle crushed tablets, as the drug may harm the male fetus. However, to our knowledge, there has not been a single reported case of birth defects caused by women handling broken or crushed finasteride tablets. The concern over handling crushed tablets may stem from the FDA policy, which assumes maximum absorption of the medication during any contact.

There is no evidence that exposure of pregnant women to finasteride via semen is a risk to the fetus. For those patients who wish to limit any potential contact of Finasteride, a condom can be worn during intercourse with a pregnant partner.

## Use in Post-Menopausal Women

A recent study was conducted to evaluate the efficacy of finasteride in post-menopausal women. After one year of use, there was no increased hair growth and the progression of thinning was not slowed. It is possible that the low DHT levels observed in post-menopausal women are responsible for the lack of significant response to finasteride, or that hair loss in this group is not related to androgens as all. The safety profile for the use of finasteride in post-menopausal women has not yet been established.

## Long-Term Benefits and Risks

The effects of finasteride are confined to areas of the scalp that are thinning, but where there is still some hair present. Finasteride does not seem to grow hair in completely bald areas. Therefore, the major benefit of finasteride seems to be in its ability to slow down or halt hair loss, or re-grow hair in parts of the scalp where the hair is thin. The long-term ability of finasteride to maintain one's hair is unknown. Results generally peak at one to two years and then decrease slightly after that.

The benefits of finasteride will stop if the medication is discontinued. Over the 2-6 months following discontinuation, the hair loss pattern will generally return to where it would have been if the medication had never been used.

Finasteride has now been in clinical use for almost 10 years. The small, but real, incidence of adverse reactions seen with finasteride underscores the fact that its actions are not entirely specific or fully understood. Only very long-term experience with this medication will determine all of its potential effects.

## Finasteride and Hair Transplantation

Finasteride can be a useful adjunct to surgical hair restoration for a number of reasons. Finasteride works best in the younger patient who may not yet be a candidate for hair transplantation. It is also less effective in the front part of the scalp, the area where surgical hair restoration can offer the greatest cosmetic improvement. It can regrow, or stabilize hair loss in the back part of the scalp where hair transplantation may not always be indicated.

If finasteride is proven safe and effective in the very long-term, it will allow the hair restoration surgeon   to create more density in the most cosmetically important areas (such as the front part of the scalp), since keeping reserves for future hair loss in other areas will be less of a concern.

## Patient Monitoring

It is recommended that men age 50 or over, should consult with their regular physician or urologist before using finasteride. It is also recommended that all men age 50 or over have a routine annual evaluation for prostate disease, regardless of whether finasteride is used. For those patients who are black and/or who have a family history of prostate disease, these recommendations would apply beginning at age 40. An evaluation may include a rectal examination, a baseline PSA test, and other exams that your physician feels are appropriate.

# 6

## WHAT IS A HAIR TRANSPLANT?

The basic concept of hair transplantation is straightforward and easily understood. The hair growing on the sides and lower part of the back of the head is permanent in most people. It persists even in advanced degrees of male pattern baldness because follicles in these locations are not subject to the deleterious affects of the hormone DHT, a byproduct of testosterone. The characteristics of the individual follicles move with them when they are transplanted. Therefore, permanent hair will remain permanent regardless of where it is transplanted, a phenomena termed "donor dominance." This is the basis of hair transplantation.

In the process of hair restoration surgery, permanent hair is redistributed to cover the areas of the head where the hair has thinned or has been lost. No new hair is actually created; existing hair is just moved around. Therefore, there is never a "net" increase in total hair volume. In spite of this, a skillfully performed hair transplant procedure can make a person "look" as though he or she has more hair, often considerably more.

The process of hair restoration is an aesthetic exercise as well as a technical feat. Re-distributing hair on a person's head is like painting a portrait. The physician should attempt to create a natural looking result that is consistent with the hair supply, the specific hair characteristics of the patient, and most important, the patient's goals.

As with other forms of cosmetic surgery, the art is at least as important as the surgical technique. The hair transplant surgeon must have a thorough understanding of human facial anatomy; good basic surgical skills and a thorough knowledge of different hair transplant techniques. The physician must know the physiology of hair in depth, and understand basic medical conditions that affect the scalp. He must be aware of, and be able to critically evaluate, new developments in the field. Finally, the specialist must study each patient carefully and tailor each procedure to the patient's unique attributes and needs.

## History

Transplantation of portions of hair-bearing skin from either animals or humans has been done with varying degrees of success since the early 1800's. However, significant modern developments in hair transplantation did not occur until the next century. In 1939, a Japanese dermatologist named Okuda first described the punch technique of hair transplantation. Dr. Okuda, working on severe burn patients, transplanted round grafts of skin containing hair follicles from the permanent hair-bearing areas into slightly smaller round openings in scarred areas of scalp. The grafts continued to produce hair in their new locations. In 1943, another Japanese dermatologist, Dr. Tamura, used 1-3 hair micrografts to restore female pubic hair. These very small micro-grafts were obtained from a single elliptical incision taken from the donor area. Interestingly, his techniques were very similar to those we are using today. The work of both of these physicians were published in Japanese medical journals, but their pioneering procedures remained unknown to the Western World because of World War II.

Hair transplantation was rediscovered by Dr. Norman Orentreich in New York City in 1952, where he performed the first hair transplant for male pattern alopecia. In 1959, Dr. Orentreich published his work in the Annals of the New York Academy of Science (after several years of rejection by a disbelieving medical community). In this publication he put forth his theory of "donor dominance" and this began the "modern" era of hair transplantation. Unfortunately, his work paralleled the "punch" technique of Okuda, rather than the "micrograft" technique of Tamura and so, by the 1960's, hair restoration surgery in the United States was off and running, but in the wrong direction.

## What is a Hair Graft?

During  hair transplant surgery, small grafts of skin containing hair follicles are removed from the areas of permanent hair in the back and on the sides of the head, and moved to the areas where balding or thinning occurs. The grafts are placed into openings created in the bald area where hair is desired. The openings can be  slits (incisions where tissue is not removed), a punch hole, or laser hole (where recipient tissue is actually removed or destroyed).  Both the size of the grafts and the size of the wounds where they are placed  have become smaller over the past 40 years. This decrease in size has made the transplants dramatically more natural in appearance.

The way the transplanted hair follicle behaves differs from most other "organ" transplants.  When kidney, heart or liver transplants are performed, the person receiving the transplant must remain on powerful immune suppressing medications to prevent rejection, as the organs are generally transplanted from one person to another.  Since a hair transplant is an "autograft," (a transplant from one part of the body to another) there is no rejection and no medications are required.

## Different Graft Sizes

Hair grafts are divided into four general categories: traditional standard grafts, minigrafts, micrografts, and follicular unit grafts.  Traditional standard grafts are 3-4 mm in diameter and have 12-30 hairs per graft. Minigrafts are smaller, 1.2-

2.5 mm in diameter, and have 4-12 hairs per graft. Micrografts are even smaller measuring 1.5-1.0 mm or less in diameter, with 1-3 hairs per graft. Follicular units are the naturally growing groups of hair follicles. Each follicular unit graft contains 1-4 hair follicles.

Although minigrafts and micrografts are a significant improvement over the larger grafts, they are not ideal. The idea was reasonable: to keep the number of hairs in each graft low. However, mini-micrografts were moved in unnatural arrangements and the naturally growing groups of hair were ignored. This is because in minigrafting and micrografting, the donor hair is harvested with a multi-bladed knife. This instrument that breaks up naturally occurring follicular units and causes unavoidable damage to follicles. Focusing on the number of hairs, rather than the naturally growing groups, minigrafting and micrografting damage the follicles, causing a significant transplant failure rate. Micrografts tend to produce a thin look when used exclusively over the entire head, and often produce inconsistent graft growth.

Follicular unit grafts are based upon the observation that hair emerges from the scalp in naturally occurring clusters called follicular units. Each follicular unit is comprised of one to four terminal hairs. By using the follicular unit as the base unit of the transplant, the surgeon can create hair patterns that mimic the way hair grows naturally. The art of the follicular unit approach is that the characteristics of the patient's hair dictate the size of the implant (rather than the doctor). The surgeon determines distribution and balance. By preserving both the natural physiologic and aesthetic elements of human hair, the best cosmetic results can be achieved.

There are many advantages of Follicular Unit Transplantation over micrografting. A fuller look is achieved, as the grafts can be of the same size (or even smaller) than micrografts yet contain more hair. Graft growth is more consistent than when the follicular units are split up. Recipient wounds heal more quickly because sites in the recipient area are smaller, and the results look more natural. Follicular unit transplantation allows the doctor to distribute grafts to mimic the way hair grows naturally in the patient's own scalp.

Follicular Unit Transplantation enables the surgeon to restore more hair using a smaller amount of donor tissue, as the technique is more efficient than minigrafting and micrografting. The tissue between the follicular groups is dissected away, while the vital support structures around the unit are preserved. Cobblestoning (irregularities in the surface of the scalp) and depigmentation (the appearance of whitish blemishes of the transplanted skin) can be avoided because excess skin in the grafts has been removed, making the grafts significantly smaller. The follicular units produce very small physiologic implants, that can, in turn, be inserted into very small sites. In addition, larger amounts of hair may be safely moved in one session reducing the necessity for multiple procedures. The patient benefits significantly with less time devoted to restoration, fewer procedures and, often, a lower cost per graft.

The large plugs used in the past, transplanted far too much bald skin in each graft. Minigrafts and micrografts also consist of multiple (partial or complete) follicular units along with the intervening skin. Even micrografts containing as few as two or three hairs may contain unnecessary skin if the hair was taken from two or more separate follicular units. Hair moved in these types of grafts results in transplanted tissue that has the same ratio of follicles to skin as the donor area. As healing occurs, the scar around the graft contracts, pushing the hairs in the graft together, and the density of the hair within the graft increases. The hair density within these larger grafts often exceeds the hair density in the donor area. This higher hair density within grafts is intrinsic to the principles of scar contraction, and produces the pluggy appearance of traditional grafts.

There are other problems associated with the use of the larger grafts. It takes four to six days for the buds of new capillary blood vessels to grow into the grafts from the surrounding tissue. Until these new blood vessels grow into the grafts, the graft's cells depend upon the surrounding tissue fluid seeping into them to bring them oxygen and nutrients. Hair follicle cells have a very high metabolic rate, and they require more oxygen and other nutrients than other cells. If the graft is too large, the cells of the follicles in the center of the graft may die before sufficient oxygen and nutrients can reach the center of the graft. The follicles at the periphery of the graft survive because they receive sufficient oxygen. When hair finally grows from these larger grafts, it has a doughnut configuration, with hair at the edges and a bald central area. This is one of the numerous reasons why many doctors have changed to the use of smaller grafts.

## Small Grafts vs. Large Grafts

To meet the demand for natural-looking hairlines, doctors began decreasing the size of grafts in the 1980s. Smaller grafts had the advantage of being less visible during the transition period after transplantation and before the hair had grown in. Large grafts placed in a frontal hairline look pluggy and unnatural when the hair was combed back or to the side. The patient in this situation was forced to comb his hair forward and down to hide his hairline. When large grafts are placed behind the hairline or in the crown, they tend to look like intermittent clumps of hair and are very difficult to disguise.

The amount of time and work needed to place a large number of tiny grafts is much greater than the time and work needed to place a smaller number of larger grafts. Smaller grafts also produce a thinner (but more natural) appearance. If the restoration process is stopped before completion, the patient will still look natural. Larger grafts tend to obligate the patient to complete multiple sessions in the quest for natural-looking results and the patient's appearance can be strikingly unnatural before the work is completed. Even with additional work, the large graft transplants often fail to appear natural because they are intrinsically clumpy. On close inspection, it is literally impossible for large graft transplants to look and feel natural, even after the best work.

Patients should discuss the size of the grafts and the planned distribution of the grafts in detail with their surgeons. Some surgeons use larger grafts for the bulk of the work and then use smaller grafts in an attempt to hide the larger grafts. Others only transplant small grafts. Some hair transplant surgeons invent unusual terms for grafts in an attempt to make it appear that they have some special, unique knowledge or technique. These terms are intended to imply special variations in graft sizes or an invisible appearance of the grafts. Do not be confused by arcane terminology. The potential patient should be wary when a doctor claims to have a unique technology or technique that no other doctor knows about or uses, unless it is documented and published in a peer-reviewed medical journal.

## Hybrid Grafting Technique

The use of larger grafts for the top and non-central portion of the crown and smaller grafts for the frontal hairline and perimeter of the transplant has a variety of names including the Hybrid Technique, Blend Grafting and Variagrafting. Although this hybrid approach is detectable on close inspection, it may not be noticeable in a social setting unless the hair is wet or the patient is in bright sunlight. The results are best in patients who have curly, white or very blonde hair. Although the look from a distance of two to three feet in soft lighting may be relatively undetectable, on closer inspection it always is; and it will never fool the barber.

In individuals with curly or wavy hair, the hybrid approach may be a reasonable way to reduce the costs of the process.

For individuals with straight hair, such an approach can be disastrous, particularly if the color of the hair stands out against   distinctly contrasting skin tones. The hybrid procedure generally costs less, and can be performed without the intense labor required for larger sessions of small grafts. The larger grafts may range from 1.5 mm in size to more than 2 mm in size. Another disadvantage for those who will accept the hybrid compromise is that the larger grafts may become more evident when further balding occurs, particularly when recession allows them to be viewed from a different angle. The hybrid approach is more a short-term economic solution than a long-term one and is not recommended by NHI physicians.

## Appearance of Hair Transplants

What makes a hair transplant bad is that everyone can tell it is a transplant. The uneven, patchy effect of the large pluggy grafts occurs when large grafts are used and the spaces between the grafts are wide. This causes a contrast between the bald skin and the islands or clumps of hair and creates a "dolls-head" appearance. Traditional hair transplants also produce small subtle deformities in the skin. Skin abnormalities with larger grafts occur for two reasons. First, the surface of the transplanted skin may not be aligned with the surface of the surrounding scalp (this is seen in larger hair grafts where the transplanted skin has enough mass to produce the problem). Second, scar contraction and/or skin dimpling occurs at the recipient site from the healing process. As the grafts increase in size, these abnormalities occur with increasing frequency. When the grafts are smaller than the critical size, these problems rarely exist.

The natural hair mass is composed of hair groupings of one to four hairs that are close together (follicular units). In nature, only single-hair follicular units appear at the leading edge of the hairline. To appear natural, a hair transplant should simulate that look as closely as possible. An ideal hair transplant consists of follicular units placed closely together with naturally occurring single units placed at the frontal edge of the hairline. When follicular grafts are placed into small sites, skin deformities are rare, or nonexistent.

## Method of Harvesting Grafts

There are four common methods of harvesting donor grafts. The original method, devised by Dr. Orentreich, used a hand punch to cut single grafts 4-mm in size that could contain up to 30 or more hairs. Each punch hole was separated by small islands of skin. Besides producing very large grafts, there was hair wastage around the periphery, due to transection and improper angling of the punch. This method is now rarely used. A second method utilizes a mechanical punch held in a small hand engine to core out a number of round grafts of known size. The punch turns at very high speeds; the torque and heat energy generated by this method will damage the donor grafts.

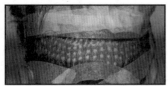

Figure 6–1. A patient who had the open donor technique. Note the Swiss cheese scarring in the area where the grafts were taken. This technique was extensively performed during the '70s and early '80s. Some surgeons still use this outmoded technique today.

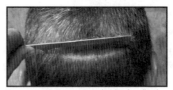

Figure 6–2. A patient who had Follicular Unit Hair Transplantation using single strip harvesting. Note that the scar is barely noticeable.

The donor grafts obtained by the punch methods can be made into minigrafts by halving or quartering them. The donor area can then be closed by suturing or can be left open. If the donor sites are not closed, they develop significant scars. Most doctors have abandoned these techniques.

The third method uses multiple, parallel scalpels attached together on a handle, called a multi-bladed knife. Multiple thin strips of hair-bearing donor skin are removed simultaneously and then grafts of the desired size are cut from the thin strips of tissue produced by the multi-bladed knife. Using a scalpel does not produce any torque or heat energy; therefore, no heat or torque damage to the grafts can occur. This method is quick and simple and still quite popular. Unfortunately, this method can cause extensive damage to the donor tissue, as it is impossible to line up the multiple blades parallel to the hair follicles. Because of this there is unacceptable cutting of individual follicles (transection) and breaking up of naturally occurring follicular units.

In a fourth method, called single strip harvesting, the donor tissue is removed as a single strip. The great advantage of this method is that the tissue is removed from the scalp with the minimal amount of "blind" cutting. The only blind cutting is the single incision around the periphery of the donor strip as it is removed. All further dissection can be then performed by direct visualization using a dissecting stereomicroscope. This keeps potential damage to follicles at an absolute minimum and allows preservation of intact naturally occurring follicular units. In order to perform Follicular Unit Transplantation, single strip harvesting and stereo-microscopic dissection must be used.

## Appearance of the Donor Area

Unless the back and side hair is extremely short, the donor area will be covered by hair and will be unnoticeable after surgery. All donor "harvests" result in a scar, but if done properly, the scars may become, for all practical purposes, virtually invisible. Not only is it important for the scar to be closed meticulously, but also the scar must be placed in the proper position, in the mid-portion of the donor area. Scars that are place too low have an increased risk of stretching from the movement of the neck muscles. Scars that are placed very high run the risk of being visible if there is extensive balding.

In addition, the hair that is obtained from these high incisions may not be permanent.

Re-harvesting the same area is important to keep visible scaring to a minimum and to keep the donor scar in the mid-portion of the permanent zone. Some doctors harvest a new area for each surgery. When many surgeries are done, these patients have a stepladder appearance of the back of the scalp from the multiple scars. Each scar distorts the hair shafts in either side of the adjacent skin. This distortion occurs because scars tend to contract. When contraction occurs, the microscopic structures around the scar are pulled. If different donor sites are chosen for each hair transplant procedure, the total area for distortion of the hair follicles becomes quite extensive. Such distortions can affect the surgeon's ability to maximize the donor hair supply for more extensive hair transplant restorations and often limit the surgeon's ability to keep the donor site undetectable. The following photographs demonstrate the contrast between extensive scarring associated with multiple procedures, when donor hair is taken from different areas for each procedure and a properly placed scar repeated from the same location.

## Scar Improvement

Hair transplant specialists are often confronted with patients whose donor areas have been severely scarred by an older harvesting method, improper harvesting techniques, too many surgeries, or, in the rare patient, a large scar due to the patient's individual healing tendencies. Frequently when scars occur, they can be surgically improved. The modification of obvious scarring may be attempted at the same time as a transplant procedure.

## Hairlines

Proper selection of donor sites and graft sizes are extremely important aspects of the surgery. Design of the hairline and placement of the recipient sites are also crucial to an aesthetically successful outcome. Some doctors create the same standard hairline on every patient. This practice is less than ideal. Natural hairlines vary from one individual to another as much as facial features do. The hair transplant specialist must be aware of the spectrum of variations that normally occur. Few natural hairlines are symmetrical; therefore, one should not attempt to create a perfectly balanced hairline, as it is distinctly unnatural looking. Men of European descent with naturally full heads of hair often have receded corners at the temple or a slightly pointed hairline. Men from the Middle East and Asia often have wide, flat hairlines with a gentler curve. Men of African descent tend to have a very straight, flat hairline.

Errors can occur when over-demanding patients or over-aggressive doctors place the hairline too low on the forehead, or restore the juvenile hairline. The patient must have an active voice in all decisions concerning the placement and design of the hairline, but it is up to the physician to educate the patient so that his decisions will be appropriate in the future as well as the present. Faulty decisions, once acted upon, will be permanent. The only remedy for a hairline that has been placed too low is to remove the grafts surgically; a situation that is better avoided than treated after the error has been made.

## Hair and Its Variations

Certain hair types may be more common in certain human groups. Understanding these characteristics may be critical in anticipating the results one can expect. African hair is very curly. This single characteristic makes African hair produce some of the best results in hair transplantation, but the dissection must be performed with extreme care to avoid damage to the curved follicles.

Most Asian hair is black, coarse and straight, making this

hair type the most difficult when striving for good reconstruction results with traditional hair transplant techniques, especially when the skin is fair. Korean hair, for example, requires very small grafts (usually one to two hairs per graft) to produce a natural look. In fair-haired Caucasians with a low contrast between hair and skin tones, hair transplant results can be spectacular, as the fair skin and blonde hair color match closely. Using only naturally occurring individual follicular units will produce natural results with all hair and skin types.

In addition to the variation of size and character of the terminal hairs in different areas of the head, hair grows in different directions in different parts of the scalp. Hair in back of the head grows backward and downward; hair in the front and top grows forward; hair on the sides of the head grows away from the middle of the head. The place where they meet in the crown is reflected in the "cowlick." The art of your surgeon should reflect knowledge of your natural growth patterns, your hairstyle preferences, and how you want your hair to look when groomed or un-groomed. To create a natural looking head of hair, the grafts that go into the recipient area should produce hair that is as close as possible in consistency and direction to the original hair and should reflect the various characteristics of both your hair and heritage.

A working knowledge of the nuances of different hair characteristics is essential in producing an ideal result. Fine techniques are necessary to make perfect donor grafts that are exactly parallel to the direction of the hair shafts of the original hair in the transplanted area. Artistry is required to design a hairline that is appropriate to the size and shape of the patient's head. Precision must be employed for the proper placement of the many small grafts.

## The Fast Track® Method

The technique of performing a large number of grafts in a single session was introduced in Brazil at the clinic of Dr.

Carlos Uebel in the mid-1980's. Work of a similar nature was performed a little later in Austria, Germany, and Japan. Dr. Uebel's focus was on moving one- to two-hair grafts in quantities of up to 1,500 grafts in a single session.

In 1992, New Hair Institute expanded upon the earlier micrograft procedures to perform large megasessions of 2,000-3,000 very small 1-3 hair grafts in a single session and called this the Fast Track® method. The procedure was popularized worldwide when, in 1994 and 1995, NHI brought several dozen live patients with their work completed to two conventions of the ISHRS (International Society of Hair Restoration Surgeons) in the United States and Canada and showed the results of these megasessions.

The results were so impressive that they put to rest the challenges to NHI's Fast Track® method and put the "Megasession" permanently on the map. In 1995, NHI began using only follicular units in these large sessions and called the procedure Follicular Transplantation. The name was formally changed to Follicular Unit Transplantation in 1998.

Although Dr. Uebel's balding patients did not necessarily have the appearance of full   heads of hair, they were able to achieve thin natural heads of hair in single sessions to frame their faces. They also had the opportunity to stop after just one session without worrying about an unfinished appearance. The Fast Track® approach takes these advances a step further and makes the transplant reconstruction fit into a socially acceptable time period. The most distinct difference between the Fast Track® and other similar transplantation procedures is the high number of hair follicles that are moved in naturally growing follicular units. This dramatically reduces the number of procedures required.

The Fast Track® method may condense the entire hair transplantation process into one or two surgical procedures. With this approach, each procedure may stand on its own, and subsequent procedures are simply the decision of the patient to add additional density or refinement. If more than one procedure is desired, another can be performed in as little as 8 months, if appropriate. A second procedure should await the results of the earlier procedure before reassessing goals and determining the cosmetic effects of the first procedure. This means that density may be added incrementally, and that the patient may stop with just one procedure if he chooses to do so and still achieve an attractive and natural outcome. With the Fast Track® method, the number of surgeries is minimized, as is the disruption of the patient's life.

# 7

# What is Follicular Unit Transplantation?

## What are Follicular Units?

Human hair grows in tiny bundles called follicular units. Although this fact had been recognized for some time by histologists (doctors who study human tissue), the existence of follicular units has been largely ignored by physicians performing hair restoration surgery.

The follicular unit of the adult human scalp consists of 1-4 terminal (full thickness) hair follicles. In areas of the scalp affected by genetic balding, the healthy terminal hairs are gradually replaced by hairs of smaller diameter and length called "miniaturized" hairs.

In addition to the full terminal hairs, the follicular unit contains 1-2 fine vellus hairs, sebaceous (oil) glands, a small muscle, tiny nerves and blood vessels, and a fine band of collagen that surrounds the unit (the perifolliculum). The follicular unit is thus the hair bearing structure of the skin and should be kept intact to insure maximum growth.

The follicular unit is seen on the surface of the scalp as a tiny group of hairs that appear to be growing together. They are best viewed under a microscope where they are seen as well-formed structures in the skin.

## What is Follicular Unit Transplantation?

Follicular Unit Transplantation is a technique, pioneered by the physicians at the New Hair Institute, in which hair is transplanted from the permanent zone in the back of the scalp

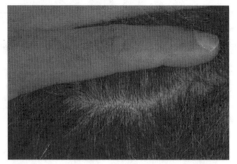

Figure 7–1. Normal scalp hair that is being parted with a hand. Note how the hair seems to grow as single strands.

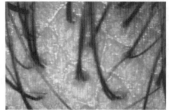

Figure 7–2. A close-up view showing the hair actually emerging in small groups called follicular units.

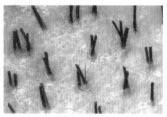

Figure 7–3. With the hair clipped, the natural hair groupings are visualized on the surface of the skin at 30x magnification through an instrument called a densitometer.

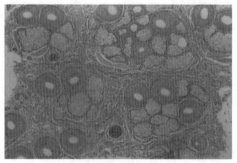

Figure 7–4. A histologic view of the corresponding follicular units seen in cross-section within the dermis.

into areas affected by genetic balding (and some other types of hair loss), using only the naturally occurring, individual follicular units. In order to remove follicular units from the back of the scalp without damaging them, the donor tissue must be removed in one piece. This technique, "single strip harvesting," is an essential component of follicular unit transplantation as it not only preserves the follicular units, but also prevents damage (transection) to the individual hair follicles. It differs dramatically from the minigrafting and micrografting technique of using a multi-bladed knife that breaks up follicular units and causes unacceptable levels of transection of hair follicles.

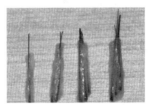

Figure 7–5. Perfectly intact 1-, 2-, 3-, and 4-hair follicular units removed from the donor strip using a dissecting stereomicroscope.

Another essential component of Follicular Unit Transplantation is "stereomicroscopic dissection." In this technique all of the follicular units are removed from the donor tissue under total microscopic control to avoid damage. Complete stereomicroscopic dissection has been shown to produce an increased yield (as much as 30%) of both the absolute number of follicular units, as well as the total amount of hair. (This procedure differs from minigrafting and micrografting in which  grafts are cut using minimal or no magnification.)

A major advantage of follicular unit transplantation (besides preserving follicular units and maximizing growth) is that it allows the surgeon to use small recipient sites. Grafts

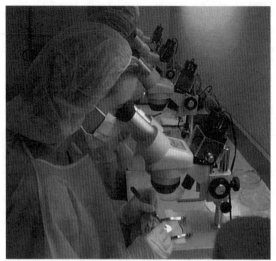

Figure 7–6. An NHI team performing stereo-microscopic dissection.

comprised of individual follicular units are small because follicular units are small, and because the surrounding non-hair bearing tissue is removed under the microscope is not transplanted. Follicular unit grafts can be inserted into tiny needle-sized sites in the recipient area, that heal in just a few days, without leaving any marks.

When performed by a skilled surgical team, Follicular Unit Transplantation can produce totally natural-looking hair transplants that maximize the yield from the patient's donor supply to give the best possible cosmetic results. Because the tiny follicular unit grafts (and the very small wounds they are placed in) allow large number of grafts to be safely transplanted in one procedure, the total restoration can be completed in the fewest possible sessions.

## The Reason for Using Only Follicular Units

The fact that scalp hair grows in follicular units, rather than individually, is most easily observed by densitometry, a simple technique whereby scalp hair is clipped short in a very

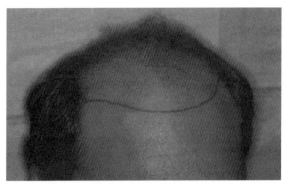

Figure 7–7. A Norwood class 6 patient with position of new hairline marked just prior to surgery.

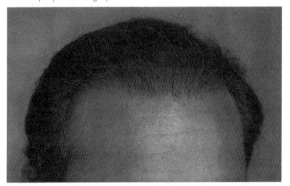

Figure 7–8. Results after two sessions of Follicular Unit Transplantation. Note the perfectly natural appearance of the frontal hairline.

small area and then observed via magnification in a 10mm² field. What is very obvious when one examines the scalp by this method, is that follicular units are relatively compact, but are surrounded by substantial amounts of non–hair bearing skin. The actual proportion of non-hair bearing skin is probably on the order of 50%, so that its inclusion in the dissection (or, conversely, its removal) will have a substantial effect upon the outcome of the surgery. When multiple follicular units are used (as in minigrafting and micrografting) the additional skin that is included will adversely affect the outcome of the surgery, by necessitating larger wounds, making the healing slower and often causing irregularities of the skin surface.

A great advantage of using individual follicular units is that the wound size can be kept to a minimum, while at the same time maximizing the amount of hair that can be placed into it. Having the flexibility to place up to 4 hairs in a tiny recipient site has important implications for the design and overall cosmetic impact of the surgery. This is one major advantage that follicular unit transplantation has over extensive micrografting. Follicular Unit Transplantation can minimize or eliminate the "see through" look that is so characteristic of micrografting.

The main reason for transplanting only individual follicular units is to duplicate the way hair naturally grows. By mimicking the way hair grows in nature, the doctor can insure that the transplant will look totally natural. Any grouping larger than the naturally occurring follicular unit will run the risk of a pluggy, tufted look.

## The Importance of Keeping Recipient Sites Small

Using only follicular units enables the recipient sites to be kept very small. In fact, in Follicular Unit Transplantation, the sites are so small that they are made with specialized instruments that are the size of 18-20 gauge needles. This is about the size that is used in routine blood tests.

The importance of minimizing the wound size in any surgical procedure cannot be over emphasized. This, of course, includes hair transplantation as well. The effects of recipient wounding impact many aspects of the surgery. Larger wounds tend to injure larger blood vessels and although the blood supply of the scalp is extensive, the damage to these vessels can have a deleterious impact on blood flow to the tissues.

Especially when transplanting large numbers of grafts per session, it is important to keep the recipient wounds as small as possible so that growth will be maximized. The compact follicular unit is the ideal way to permit the use of the smallest possible recipient site, and has made the transplantation of large numbers of grafts technically feasible. Another important advantage of the small wound is a factor that can be referred to as the "snug fit." A follicular unit graft is so small that it can always fit into a tiny wound without having to remove tissue. Unlike the punch, which destroys recipient collagen and elastic tissue, a small incision, made with a needle, retains the basic elasticity (recoil) of the recipient site. When a properly fitted graft is inserted, the recipient site will then hold it snugly in place. This "snug fit" has several advantages. During surgery, it minimizes popping and the need for the sometimes traumatic re-insertion or re-positioning of grafts. After the procedure, it ensures maximum contact of the graft with the surrounding tissue, so that oxygenation can be quickly re-established. In addition, by eliminating empty space around the graft, microscopic clots are minimized and wound healing is facilitated.

It is important to note that when trying to place larger grafts (either round or linear), into a small site (kept small to minimize tissue injury) compression of the grafts is an undesirable consequence, and may result in a tufted appearance. In contrast, when transplanting follicular units, there are no adverse cosmetic effects of compression, since follicular units are already tightly compacted structures.

Finally, large wounds cause a host of other cosmetic problems including dimpling, pigmentary alteration, depression or elevation of the grafts, or a thinned, atrophic look. The key to a natural appearing hair transplant is to have the hair emerge from perfectly normal skin. The only way to ensure this is to keep the recipient wounds small.

## How is Follicular Unit Transplantation Different from Mini-Micrografting?

This is one of the most commonly asked questions and it

is a very important one for those deciding which hair restoration procedure to choose. In contrast to Follicular Unit Transplantation, where the graft sizes are determined by nature, in mini-micrografting (the combination of minigrafts and micrografts as defined in Chapter 6) the graft sizes are arbitrarily determined by the doctor who cuts the donor tissue into the size pieces that he wants. Another name for this technique is mini-micrografts "cut to size."

In mini-micrografting, neither preserving follicular units, nor even keeping hair follicles intact, are felt to be that important. Rather, the speed and economics of the procedure are the deciding factors. Mini-micrografters use a multi-bladed knife to quickly generate thin strips of tissue and then use direct visualization (rather than microscopic control) to cut the tissue. The resulting grafts are generally larger than follicular units and since the excess skin is not trimmed away the donor sites (wounds) are also larger.

It should be apparent from the comparison shown on the next page that Follicular Unit Transplantation is superior in producing a natural, undetectable result, in maximizing healing, and preserving precious donor hair. Mini-micrografting, however, requires a smaller staff and each procedure is cheaper and shorter (although in the end it takes more procedures and therefore may cost just as much for this technique).

For more detailed information on NHI's Follicular Unit Transplantation, please see the reference section in the back of the book. Many of the original articles can be found on our web site www.newhair.com in the section, NHI Medical Publications.

The following table summarizes the major differences between Follicular Unit Transplantation and Mini-Micrografting:

| | **Follicular Unit Transplantation** | Vs | **Mini-Micrografting** |
|---|---|---|---|
| **THE GRAFTS** | | | |
| Follicular Units used exclusively | Yes | | No |
| Graft size | Uniformly small | | Larger |
| Number of hairs per graft | 1-4 | | 1-6 (or more) |
| Hair/skin ratio in graft | High | | Average |
| Extra skin transplanted | No | | Yes |
| Wound size | Uniformly small | | Variable |
| | | | |
| **THE TECHNIQUE** | | | |
| Harvesting type | Single-Strip | | Multi-bladed knife |
| Microscopes required | Yes | | No |
| Follicular Units Preserved | Yes | | No |
| Follicular transection | No | | Yes |
| Maximizes donor supply | Yes | | No |
| | | | |
| **THE RESULTS** | | | |
| Healing time | Fast | | Slower |
| Skin surface change | No | | Yes |
| Maximum fullness | Yes | | No |
| Undetectable | Yes | | No |
| | | | |
| **COST & CONVENIENCE** | | | |
| Staff requirements | Moderate | | Small |
| Duration of individual procedure | Long | | Short |
| Time for complete restoration | Short | | Long |
| Cost per procedure | More | | Less |
| Total cost for restoration | Similar | | Similar |

# 8

# YOUR MASTER PLAN FOR FUTURE HAIR LOSS

Hair restoration is as much an art form as a medical discipline and is best planned, performed, and completed by the same surgeon or surgeons trained in using the same techniques. If various surgeons work on the same patient and different techniques are employed, the results may look more like a patchwork quilt than a normal head of hair. As with great artists, the best surgeons work from a Master Plan. They sketch out a plan, project the amount of work needed, and then implement the plan. In contrast to art, in which the artist has sole discretion in how the work is created, both the doctor and the patient must assess the soundness of a Master Plan in a hair restoration process.

If the patient feels the proposed Master Plan is inconsistent with his or her goals or the course is not consistent with his or her expectations, then the patient should tell the doctor about his or her concerns. The patient should always feel comfortable enough to speak his or her mind and expect the doctor to react responsively. Your doctor should have your best interests in mind, and answer your questions directly. After the work has been done, it is common for fear and uncertainty to set in while one waits for the hair to grow in and the final picture to unfold. It is important for the physician to be supportive and accessible during this period as well.

Physicians who perform general surgery need little artistic talent to perform what is, most often, a technical process. In hair transplants, as in other forms of cosmetic surgery, the work is completely visible. Although the technical demands of a hair transplant can be substantial, particularly when done in large numbers, there is no substitute for the skill and experience of the surgeon in laying out the Master Plan, including creating the hairline, and blending the various hair characteristics. The artistic ability of the surgeon is best appreciated by seeing, first hand, the results of his or her work.

## The Course of Hair Loss

Most male hair loss is a progressive process in which a person's full head of hair inexorably changes to a thinning or receding state and finally to a balding state. It is common to see the effects of genetic balding in young men start when they are in their late teens or early 20's. When hair loss occurs early it can be rapid and quite extensive. More commonly, it is a slow progression, in which the significant hair loss occurs over a 10-20 year period. The process can start at any age, possibly even in a person in his 50's. In the entire male population, slightly over one-third experience significant balding by the time they reach their 40's. Fewer than one in eight men become extensively bald (have only a wreath of hair around the sides and back of the head) by the age of 80.

Genetic hair loss also affects women, but the process rarely leads to the type of extensive recession or balding frequently seen in men. In genetic hair loss for either sex, the process accelerates as a person ages and frequently does so in waves rather than in a continuous fashion. Stress seems to accelerate short-term loss, but rarely affects the long-term course. There are periods between the cycles where the hair loss stops for a time (these periods can be very lengthy in women), but progression is inevitable in all those genetically predisposed.

Drugs, like minoxidil (Rogaine), may slow the balding process, but are unsuccessful in completely averting hair loss. Newer medications, such as finasteride (Propecia) seem to be more successful in preventing further hair loss on a long-term basis. These drugs may successfully be combined with surgical hair restoration.

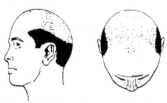

Figure 8–1. Typical Permanent Hair Zone

## An Individualized Master Plan

Each person is born with a limited supply of hair. Much of the hair around the side and back of the head may be considered permanent in that it is genetically programmed to last well into a person's senior years. This permanent area of hair, commonly called the "donor area", is where the hair is taken when a transplant is performed. Hair not located in this region may be susceptible to the genetic balding process. All surgical hair restoration procedures move hair from the donor area to areas where the hair is not permanent in genetically affected people. The permanent hair may be thought of as a "bank" from which withdrawals are possible, but to which no deposits can be made.

The need for a Master Plan individualized for each patient is critical because each person has a unique combination of hair density, hair character, hair color, skin color, balding pattern, age and genetic characteristics. In this chapter, we will describe the hair loss patterns and hair restoration plans of several patients with various balding patterns. By studying the specific case histories, you may gain further insight into your own situation. Although this book will enable you to gain an understanding of the hair restoration process and the importance of your Master Plan.

Only an experienced and honest hair restoration physician can customize your Master Plan to meet your unique needs. Over the past 30+ years, this industry has not been forthcoming and open in its representations of the results obtained from the various hair restoration procedures. Much of the lack of openness still exists. For this reason, the buyer should be wary of dubious medical claims and patient results that cannot be confirmed.

## The Donor Hair Bank

The average Caucasian is born with approximately 100,000 hairs on the head. Those of Asian and African descent are generally born with lower densities. If we were to look at the Norwood Class 7 hair loss pattern as the final stage of hair loss (illustration above), up to 75% of these hairs, or 75,000 will be lost and 25,000 hairs will remain (permanent hair) in the donor area. A portion of this permanent hair can be utilized for hair transplantation. A standard rule of thumb is that, in a person with average hair density, one can deplete the permanent zone by approximately 50% to 12,500 hairs. Thus, in this Class 7 male, it is generally possible to move some 12,500 hairs or, assuming a normal distribution of one, two, three and four-hair follicular unit, approximately 5,000-6,000 follicular unit grafts can be moved.

If the density in the donor area is high (a person born with 150,000 hairs), the amount of usable donor hair increases significantly. In a person born with 150,000 hairs and in an advanced stage of balding, the donor areas would contain 37,000 hairs (instead of 25,000 hairs in the average person). Leaving the required 12,500 hairs in the donor area means that there are some 25,000 hairs available for transplant. Note that a 50% increase in hair density results in a 100% increase in available donor hair. Unfortunately, the reverse is also true. Suppose the patient has 75,000 hairs at birth. This means he will have 20,000 hairs in the donor area leaving only 7,500 hairs for transplant. Thus, a 25% reduction in hair density results in a 50% reduction in available donor hair.

The other key factor affecting the mathematics of the Master Plan involves scalp laxity (the flexibility and looseness of the scalp). This measurement is a factor in determining the size of the donor area that may be safely removed in a single surgical procedure and will determine the total amount of movable hair long-term.

In a patient with a tight scalp, it may be relatively easy to harvest the needed grafts in the first procedure. However, in subsequent sessions, the tight scalp may become a significant limiting factor. Such a patient may eventually be able to move the needed amount of donor hair, but may require several procedures to accomplish this goal. More commonly, the total amount of movable hair is reduced in patients with tight scalps and it is important for the physician to identify this before the surgery is begun so that a realistic long-term master plan can be established. Certainly, many patients with tight scalps have very successful transplants, but the expectations of having full coverage might be unrealistic.

For a single surgical procedure, more hair can be moved when the scalp is loose and the density is high. Usually in subsequent procedures, scalp laxity returns to its original state, but eventually it may tighten to reduce the yield with subsequent procedures. If the laxity returns to its preoperative state, a similar area can be moved once again, but the density of the hair in that portion of the scalp will be less, as the skin will have stretched to accommodate the portion previously removed.

It is important to take into account both hair density and scalp laxity when we consider the amount of hair that needs to be moved. A bald scalp in the average Class 6 patient is about 80 square inches (200 cm²). A maximum of approximately 12 square inches (30 cm²) may be moved from the donor area at one time, with 9 square inches (24 cm²) being the amount removed in the average large case of Follicular Unit Transplantation. If a strip of 9 square inches will have to cover an area of some 80 square inches, if uniformly spaced, this will produce a density of approximately 12% of the original hair density. This may not seem like a lot, but if planned properly, the density achieved in the front part of the scalp can be significantly increased due to the forward weighting of sites (making them closer together towards the front) and graft sorting (using larger naturally occurring follicular units in the forelock area). Aesthetic manipulations of graft placement, performed by experienced hair restoration surgeons can make dramatic differences in the outcome of the surgery and enable an entire restoration to be completed in a limited number of sessions. From an aesthetic perspective, gains from subsequent procedures produce a less dramatic change, but they have the ability to significantly increase fullness. Thickening a thin head of hair is less noticeable than going from a balding to a thinning appearance, but is very important to getting the maximum benefit from your restoration.

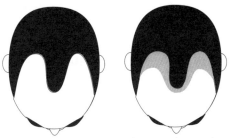

Figure 8–2. Before and After Procedure. Since the treated area is minimal, the new density in the transplanted area may be closer to the original density than when the hair transplant covers a more extensive area.

At the other end of the spectrum, in a person with early hair loss (a Norwood Class 3 for example) who simply wanted to fill in the corners of his hairline to cover an area of 4 square inches, it would be easy to move a piece of donor scalp from the permanent zone close to the size of the area to be covered. The new density of this treated area would be much closer to the original density than the previous example. The most important issue, however, is to project the future needs of the patient to make sure that sufficient donor hair remains to address the evolving balding pattern. Great care must be taken so that excessive amounts of hair are not removed from the donor area to treat the limited recession, given the possibility that such a patient may need to reserve his donor hair to cover evolving hair loss.

The average range of follicular unit grafts used per session at the New Hair Institute is from 600 (for early balding) to 2,400 (for Class 6 and 7 patients). The average case performed at the New Hair Institute for all stages of balding (all Norwood Classes) is around 1,500 follicular unit grafts. Since there is approximately one follicular unit per mm$^2$ in the scalp, a case of 1,500 follicular units would require 1,500 mm$^2$ of tissue or 15cm$^2$, providing that none of the donor hair is wasted. A recent retrospective study at the New Hair Institute, which reviewed cases performed using "single strip harvesting" and "stereo-microscopic dissection" showed this to be the case. In the average patient, 1 cm$^2$ of donor tissue yielded 100 follicular unit grafts, exhibiting virtually no wastage.

Some patients express concern about the size of the donor strip that needs to be harvested from the back of the scalp. In Follicular Unit Transplantation, a 1,500 graft case would require only a single 1cm wide by 15 cm long strip of donor tissue. This is just slightly larger than the size of a pen.

When considering the donor supply, the most important question for the patient to ask is "will the technique used to harvest and transplant hair minimize wastage, so that the maximum degree of fullness may be obtained from a specific amount of donor hair?" As discussed in Chapter 7, the answer to the question is that the physician must employ the technique of "single strip harvesting" when removing the donor tissue followed by "stereo-microscopic dissection" into individual follicular unit grafts if maximum use of the donor hair supply is to be achieved.

## Aesthetics: The Bottom Line

Restoring your hairline, or increasing the appearance of

fullness, is not purely a reflection of the amount of hair moved, or the number of grafts transplanted. There is an art in the design of the surgical process that is critical in producing an aesthetically pleasing result. Some of us are better hair transplant candidates (more hair, better color, thicker hair shafts, wavier hair); these factors produce more fullness and better coverage with a smaller quantity of follicular unit grafts.

It is tempting to try to reduce the Master Plan to a matter of numbers, but that would be inappropriate. For example, a doctor tells patient that he needs to move 10,000 hairs in 1,000 grafts in four divided sessions of 250 grafts each. The patient wants to compare the medical recommendations and prices at various clinics, but when he visits the clinics, he receives a mind-numbing array of contradictory information on prices. He hears about short cuts such as scalp reductions that are represented (falsely) as a way to save hair for future transplant work.

Once the hair has grown in, the achieved fullness and the detailed appearance of the hairline will be a reflection of many factors, including the number of hairs transplanted, the distribution of the transplanted hair, and the method of styling used after the hair grows in. There is no substitute for a natural look. After one is comfortable that the physician will efficiently utilize the donor hair without wastage, the next most important question for the person to ask is "How natural will the transplant appear throughout the growing phase and how natural will the hair transplant look after the restoration is complete?"

If the doctor moves 10,000 hairs in 1,000 grafts averaging 10 hairs each in a checkerboard pattern, the result may appear full, but it will have a "doll's head" appearance. Grafts of 10 or more hairs each (or any graft containing more hair groupings than normally found in his head) may take a long time to heal and the skin often assumes a cobblestone appearance with a white-scarred base. This type of change is permanent. Even if camouflaged by a hairline of finer, smaller grafts, the plugs will be visible whenever the hair is wet or anytime careful styling is not possible. The prospective patient must be careful when he is viewing advertisement photographs. Photographs often do not show the hairline up close, without careful styling or when it is wind-blown or wet. If you meet the patient, you can see what the photograph may not show.

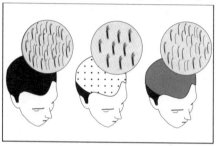

Figure 8–3. Comparison of natural hair density (left), pluggy appearance (center) and NHI coverage (right).

As an alternative to the 1,000 ten-hair grafts, the doctor could transplant 10,000 donor hairs in their naturally occurring follicular units. In a patient with 2.3 hairs per follicular unit, this would translate to 4,300 follicular unit grafts, averaging 2.3 hairs each. With NHI's Fast Track® method, this can be accomplished in two sessions.

Since the graft is small and reproduces the one, two, three and four-hair groupings that naturally appear in a person's scalp, the grafts are virtually undetectable, whether the hair is carefully styled or mussed by wind, water, or one's significant other. The overall density in the transplanted area may be the same in both the 10-hair graft example and the two-hair graft example, but in the case of smaller grafts, the surgeon can carefully place the follicles in a way that mimics nature, thus allowing a person to groom his hair the way he chooses.

As a hair transplant patient, you must be in control of what happens to you, especially in the size, the number and the distribution of the transplants. You should be able to control your hairstyle; that hairstyle may be significant in your hair transplantation. With small grafts weighted to the front or on the parted side, styling the hair straight back or combing it from the side produces a layering effect which makes the hair appear fuller and thicker. Layering is a critical element in the aesthetics of the hair restoration process, and it becomes increasingly important as the balding pattern progresses.

It is important to consider other elements related to the aesthetics of coverage, such as hair type and skin color. For a person with blonde or white hair and light skin, fewer hairs need to be moved to produce the illusion of fullness than in a person with black hair and a fair skin. A blonde, wavy haired person can lose 70% of the hair on the top of the head and not look bald because of the aesthetics of color, contrast and layering. An "afro" on a person with dark skin will produce more fullness than an Asian's black straight hair on light skin. Bleaching the hair or adding white, gray, silver or blonde streaks can add the appearance of fullness to those who are thinning. Such color alterations tend to inhibit the eye's ability to discriminate the details of the balding or thinning process. The doctor and patient must design a personalized hair restoration Master Plan that will be aesthetically pleasing for the patient, throughout his life. All of the following elements are critical in this process:

- Current balding pattern,
- Projected hair loss,
- Hair density,
- Hair and skin color,
- Thickness of each hair shaft,
- Hair character: straight, wavy, or wiry, and
- Scalp laxity.

To illustrate the complexity of predicting the final appearance, two examples are presented. Both patients received about 3,500 grafts and had advanced balding patterns.

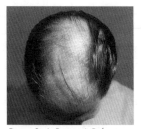

Figure 8–4. Patient A Before Surgery.

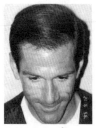

Figure 8–5. After one procedure.

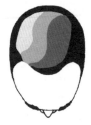

Figure 8–6. Diagrammic representation of layering

Patient A's transplant is weighted to the front and the left side where his natural part originates (see image on the right). He prefers to keep his hair long, and it is of average thickness. His hair is groomed carefully and styled to layer from the part side across the front. When hair can be styled like this, it gives the best coverage (just like a thatched roof protects a house from rain). By layering the hair, the light does not pass through the scalp hair easily, so the lower transplanted density appears more full.

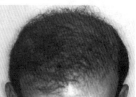

Figure 8–7. Patient B. Uniformly distributed transplanted hair in a patient who was very bald. The very short hair precludes layering and gives a see-through appearance.

Patient B's transplant is distributed more uniformly over the scalp. He has shorter hair that tends to stand up rather than layer from side to side. As the hair stands up, the light penetrates through the hair to the scalp more easily and making the lower density more apparent. Patient B prefers to keep his hair short; it does not exceed one inch at any point. Since his hair is finer and curlier than Patient A, the amount of hair available to cover the scalp is less. In addition, Patient B does not take advantage of his curly hair because he chooses to keep it short.

## Setting Realistic Expectations

While each patient's healing and hair growth profile will dictate the actual course of the post-operative period, it is important to understand the differences seen in patients with different hair characteristics. All prospective patients should view the finished work of people who have had a transplant. No two people are alike; therefore, two hair loss patterns require a different amount of work, hair distribution and budget. It is critical that hair transplant candidates make their own assessment of the process with a physician who works with them to establish realistic expectations.

Your physician should have appropriate instruments to measure hair density. The ability to measure the density of a person's hair, tells us about the "working material" the surgeon can expect to use in the reconstruction over time. A house builder would not want to design a house without having enough lumber to complete the job. The surgeon should address a similar issue, for to put together a well-designed Master Plan, the surgeon must scientifically estimate the amount of available donor hair.

The hair population of the normal human scalp in a non-balding individual is between 60,000 - 200,000 hairs. Each square inch of scalp reflects a density consistent with the overall population. If one's hair population is on the lower end of the scale, the available hair for transplantation is more limited. If one's hair population is on the high end of the scale, many possibilities exist. Be wary of surgeons who run their hands through the donor area, and comment: "you have lots of hair." Most patients want to believe such statements and this can result in unrealistic expectations for the results of the transplant. By measuring the supply of the donor area, both doctor and patient can be confident in a design for hair replacement that is unlikely to go awry.

## The Frontal Hairline

In the majority of patients, establishing the frontal hairline is the most important function of the first procedure. The frontal hairline should frame the face and restore a balance to the patient's facial proportions in a way that is appropriate for a mature individual. It should not be a low, teenage hairline. The common practice of creating a high hairline with the intention of lowering it in a subsequent procedure should be avoided, since each procedure then becomes as visible as the one before it. In addition, the surgeon doesn't have the advantage of using the second procedure to increase the density of the first.

If the intent is to conserve hair in anticipation of a very limited donor supply, one could still maximize the cosmetic impact of the surgery by creating more recession at the temples or not extending the transplant as far back towards the crown. However, the position of the mid-portion of the frontal hairline (the "forelock" region) should not be compromised, as this defines the look of the individual. Creating a hairline too high (in the hope of conserving donor hair) only accentuates the patient's baldness by enlarging the forehead and distorting the normal facial proportions.

The practice of placing hair behind an existing hairline was very popular when plugs were used. Early on, the patient's existing hair could soften the appearance of grafts that were too large to stand on their own. However, as the old hairline recedes, a new procedure in this area would be visible, as the proper hairline would still have to be established.

When surgery is performed when adequate frontal hairline coverage is still present, any benefit of increased fullness behind the frontal hairline may be more than offset by the acceleration of hair loss from the procedure and the risk of disrupting a hairline that might have persisted for a number of years longer. Therefore, a patient should be skeptical when a surgeon recommends surgery with a good frontal hairline already present and with little thinning overall.

To allow for very close placement of the grafts in the frontal hairline, NHI has developed the skills and techniques that allow for the placement of follicular unit grafts into very small recipient sites. Close placement of grafts in the frontal hairline restores the natural transition zone of the frontal hairline in a greater density than previously possible. The very small grafts also preserve more of the anatomical integrity of the scalp and blood supply at the recipient sites. Very close placement of the grafts makes it possible to complete a frontal hairline in one to two sessions.

## Covering the Crown

Crown coverage should not be a goal of the first session unless the donor hair supply is adequate. Performing crown work can be addressed after the front and top of the scalp have been adequately transplanted in those with a questionable or marginal donor supply. Since the front and top of the scalp is a single cosmetic unit, the transplant may stop after this area has been treated. The patient can then evaluate the adequacy of coverage from this procedure, and if he desires more fullness or greater density, a second session can be performed. If crown coverage is attempted in the first session, the patient's options will be much more limited and the ability to produce an aesthetically balanced transplant might be permanently eliminated.

An exception would be patients who are over the age of 30, have little apparent risk of becoming extensively bald, and who have good donor density and scalp laxity. In these individuals, transplanting the crown in the first session can provide modest coverage to the area and will serve to camouflage a limited amount of further crown balding. What should be avoided in these patients is the risky practice of repeatedly transplanting hair into the crown to achieve a high degree of density, as this density can often not be supported as the balding progresses.

## When Will A Second Session Be Needed?

Working on a scalp that has never received a hair transplant has many advantages. Grafts can be placed more easily, more securely, and closer together, since the blood supply and elasticity of the connective tissue are intact. In the donor area, maximum density and scalp mobility, as well as the absence of scarring, facilitate a fine closure. To take advantage of these factors, as many of the patient's goals should be addressed in the first procedure as possible. Often, however, a second session is required with the most common goal of increasing the density of the first.

It is important at the outset to discuss the likelihood, frequency, and cost of subsequent transplant sessions. As discussed above, a second session may be more likely in light skinned patients with dark hair, in those patients with fine hair and in those patients with straight hair (particularly when there is dark hair/light skin color contrast). In addition, a second procedure may be desirable in very bald patients with low donor density and/or reduced scalp laxity, as these factors limit the amount of hair that can be harvested at any one time. In these situations, anticipating a second surgery in the near future is a critical part of the initial planning, unless the patient is willing to accept a thinner look. A second procedure should also be anticipated from the outset in younger patients who are early in the balding process with an evolving hair loss pattern, when hair loss is rapid, and in all patients whose balding does not appear to be stable.

A special situation exists when transplanting patients with a persistent frontal forelock. The density of a forelock is often close to the patient's original frontal density, making it impractical to place additional hair into this area. Although the forelock tends to be very tenacious in some families, it still may show a slow rate of loss. If lost, a gap would be left in the central portion of the frontal hairline, making a second procedure necessary.

## Goals for the Second Session

The most common reason one plans a second procedure is to enhance the appearance of fullness. Although follicular units may have been placed as close as possible in the first session, after healing has occurred, additional units can usually be added between the first grafts. Another reason for a second session is to follow the progression of the hair loss. This is often performed in conjunction with increasing the fullness of the previously transplanted areas. Usually at the second session, more density is added to the cosmetically critical front and top of the scalp; the transplant is then extended further back to compensate for hair loss that has occurred since the first procedure or to add further areas of coverage, knowing the front and top are secure.

A third goal of the second session is to further refine the hairline. If the frontal hairline was properly placed in the first procedure, major changes in the hairline should not be necessary. However, subtle adjustments in the hairline are often performed during the second session. These refinements include: making the frontal hairline more dense, increasing the irregularity of the transition zone, flattening the hairline or blunting the corners, lowering the hairline, establishing a widow's peak, or restoring the temples.

The main decision for the second session is whether to transplant the crown, for once treatment of the area has begun, it can place significant demands upon the donor supply. Many insightful patients who are significantly bald realize that crown coverage is not realistic and are satisfied using styling techniques in conjunction with creatively distributed transplants to maximize coverage in the lightly or non-transplanted areas. This is especially true in older patients. On the other hand, a substantial number of people are very bothered by their bald crown; these patients may be devastated when hair loss occurs in the front. For most, crown balding is much less important when compared to the prospect of losing frontal hair, the entire frame of the face. Crown balding or thinning is also likely to become more acceptable as the patient ages (as will his hair loss overall). The physician then must be able to assist the patient in setting priorities that will be appropriate over the long term.

If extensive balding is likely and there is only a modest donor supply, it is usually best to treat the crown as an extension of the top, rather than as an isolated region, to ensure that the patient will not be short of donor hair. This is the reason that the treatment of the crown in a young patient should be delayed. By the second session, the surgeon is often able to assess if there is enough coverage of the front and top to attempt the crown. It is important to emphasize that when crown coverage is considered in the second session, the transplanted hair in the front and top has already been allowed to grow, so that its cosmetic impact can be assessed. The patient can thus make his own aesthetic judgments regarding whether to add additional hair to this area before transplantation of the crown is begun.

The issue of crown coverage is important because it is the least visible of the balding regions, and it has a very large surface area, producing an almost inexhaustible demand upon the donor supply. The predominantly front-to-back progression of genetic balding allows the transplanted hair to conceal hair loss behind it. More important, it is common to see a person with frontal hair and a bald area in back. Therefore, as balding continues after a transplant in the frontal area, a natural look is maintained. In contrast, the crown expands from the center outward, so that as crown balding progresses, the initially transplanted hair may become a cosmetic liability rather than an asset. This is because with further hair loss, transplantation must be continued or there will be an isolated island of hair surrounded by a moat of bald skin. In addition, the density of the normal crown increases as one moves away from the center. Thus, whatever is transplanted outward must have at least the density of the part more central to it, whereas the initial transplant of frontal hair can be followed on subsequent sessions by placing less density behind it (or not treated again). The expanding crown will always require a subsequent session of at least the same or increasing density. One way to circumvent this problem is to place "tacking hair" in the crown. These are single follicular unit grafts that function to hold down hair from the top of the scalp combed back over it, but is thin enough to not to place significant demands on the donor supply or to look unnatural if the crown expands. This technique is particularly useful in patients undergoing repair work or those with a very limited donor supply.

An important alternative to the treatment of the crown is to stop the transplant at the "vertex transition point" (the part of the scalp just in front of the swirl) and have the patient groom his hair over the non-transplanted area. This is recommended for most patients when direct crown coverage is not realistic, or when it is too early in the balding process to determine whether significant crown coverage will be possible in the future.

# 9

# How Many Grafts Will I Need?

One of the most frequent questions asked by potential hair transplant patients is: "how many grafts will I need?" The answer should:

- Take realistic expectations into consideration
- Reflect the patient's degree of hair loss, donor supply, and hair characteristics
- Be consistent with a long-term Master Plan to address future hair loss
- Address the number of potential procedures and time commitment required
- Consider the short and total long-term cost for the patient

An individual's goals must be realistic. For example, if a person has significant balding (i.e., a Norwood Class 6 or 7 pattern) and fine hair, then he should not expect a full head of transplanted hair. If he does, dissatisfaction will be inevitable. With at least 65-75% of hair lost (the typical loss in Class 6 and 7 patients), a thin head of hair is a realistic and achievable goal. Although a thin head of hair can dramatically improve patient's appearance, if he were to attempt to achieve his original density, he would run out of donor hair before the process could be completed and an unnatural appearance would result.

Working within reasonable expectations, the total number of grafts required for any one patient will depend upon hair and skin color, donor density, scalp laxity the thickness of each hair shaft, the number of hairs in each graft, and the character of the hair itself. The physician must consider these factors and the expectations of the patient in order to calculate the amount of work required. Even when these considerations are combined with the expectations of the patient, the amount of work required to make a person satisfied is sometimes difficult to predict.

Naiveté of the physician, even in those who specialize in hair transplantation, seems to be more common than many care to admit. The failure of the physician to establish realistic expectations often leads to an unhappy patient. This can only be prevented by providing a clear explanation of the hair restoration process, and specifically defining the benefits that the patient may expect to achieve.

## Hair Color and Skin Color Contrast

Hair color and its contrast to skin color is one of the most significant factors that dictate the amount of work required for hair restoration. The lower the contrast, the fewer grafts are required. Blonde hair against fair skin and dark hair against dark skin are two examples of hair combinations that produce excellent results with less work on the part of the physician (and less cost for the patient). Dark hair against pale skin often requires the most hair in the restoration process. Of course, a patient can simply lighten his hair to make the restoration look more full. One of the (few) benefits of aging is that it will accomplish reduced contrast between hair and skin all by itself.

## Hair Character

Hair character is the second most important factor in determining the amount of hair restoration work needed. Curly or wavy hair produces a full appearance more easily than straight hair. African American hair in particular curls so that a single hair shaft covers more scalp with less hair length than straight hair. Strong, naturally curly hair that holds its shape tends to produce fuller results more easily than thin straight hair that falls flat against the scalp.

## Hair Bulk

Hair bulk, or hair shaft diameter, contributes greatly to the visual impact of hair. Coarse hair has greater bulk and requires fewer hair follicles per square inch than fine hair to produce the same effect. Coarse hair usually grows naturally in smaller groups (follicular units) than fine hair and should be transplanted that way for the most natural results.

## Hair Density

In the majority of patients who are candidates for a hair transplant, hair density (the number of hairs per $cm^2$) varies from about 150 hairs/$cm^2$ to over 300 hairs/$cm^2$, with the average of about 200 hair/$cm^2$. However, as previously mentioned, hair in the human scalp does not grow as single hairs, but in groups of 1-4 hairs. Interestingly, these naturally occurring groups (called follicular units (FU)) have a relatively constant density in the scalp of 100 FU/$cm^2$. This means that the average follicular unit will contain from 2.0 hairs. Those patients who average 1.5 hairs per follicular unit will have a naturally thin appearance and therefore a thinner appearing transplant. Those patients who average 3.0 hairs per follicular unit (300/hairs per $cm^2$) will have a fuller looking transplant.

## How Many Grafts Will Make Me Happy?

When patients ask how many grafts it will take to make them happy, what they are really saying is, "give me back what I lost and I'll be happy." When this is the case, what the bald man really wants is unrealistic; therefore, one must address how much work needs to be done to make the patient satisfied. Satisfaction should be addressed in relative terms to make this problem understandable.

A man who is accustomed to his balding will be easier to please, and will accept a less full appearance than a young man who is starting to lose his hair and who remembers the days when he looked in the mirror and saw the vibrant, full hair of a teenager. The young patient wants his adolescent hairline and density back and will often be satisfied with nothing less. Since surgery is permanent, the hair-restoring surgeon must plan a hairline that will be appropriate for the patient's entire life and he must transplant a density that is consistent with long-term donor reserves. Because of these factors, some young patients are not good candidates for surgery.

The older patient with significant hair loss, on the other hand, will often be ecstatic with his mature hairline restored and a modest amount of natural-looking hair covering his head for the first time in years. For the majority of patients between these two extremes, the physician's careful guidance will help the patient understand what goals can realistically be achieved and whether hair restoration will be worthwhile.

With an understanding of human nature, hair dynamics, and practical issues, NHI has concluded that it is not always wise to recommend a specific number of grafts as though this number is an absolute amount. Instead, NHI often recommends transplant sessions of the greatest number of grafts that can be reasonably and safely moved within the confines of four important constraints listed below.

1. The patient's goals;
2. The projected pattern of hair loss in a worst-case scenario, as determined by heredity, age and physical examination;
3. The amount of hair in the permanent zone (donor area) that can be safely transplanted (this is related to a number of physical factors including donor density and scalp laxity and should be assessed by the doctor at the time of consultation); and
4. Economic and time constraints of the patient.

## NHI's Goal and Your Goal

Our goal is to help the patient understand how close he or she can come to meeting personal needs and expectations, how much the hair restoration will cost, and how many sessions it is likely to require. Do not start the hair restoration process unless you understand what it will take to finish it. With proper planning, satisfaction is easy to achieve.

Keep in mind that the transplantable hair numbers generally reflect an average amount of total hair that can be moved and applied to one's hair loss. This movable hair can be transplanted in one or multiple sessions depending on the four factors above and your doctor's skill and experience. For example, if procedures are limited to only 100 grafts each, then patients will be committed to an extended number of surgical sessions. Possibly not obvious at the onset, such extended treatment sessions often end with the patient losing interest. Financial or personal reasons may also cause the patient to fail to complete the treatment course. Just as important, multiple, small procedures move hair inefficiently and waste precious donor supply.

As discussed in Chapter 8, the impact of the transplant depends both upon the distribution of grafts as the absolute number used. Nonetheless, it is still useful for the patient anticipating surgery to have a general idea of the numbers required, both for the initial procedure and for subsequent sessions.

## What NHI Recommends

Although there is significant variation from person to person, the average number of follicular units that we generally transplant in the first session for specific Norwood classifications is listed below. We first presented these numbers in our landmark 1995 publication "Follicular Transplantation." The recommend numbers have changed little over the years, except that with the implementation of stereomicroscopic dissection, we rarely need to transplant more than 2400 grafts in a single session. All "units" or "grafts" in this discussion refer to follicular units, not minigrafts or micrografts.

## First Follicular Unit Transplantation Session

| Norwood Class | Follicular Units | Total Units With Crown |
|---|---|---|
| 3 | 800-1000+ | --- |
| 3 Vertex | 800-1000+ | 1100-1300+ |
| 3A | 1300-1600+ | --- |
| 4 | 1100-1400+ | 1500-1800+ |
| 4A | 1700-2100+ | --- |
| 5 | 1500-1800+ | 1900-2400+ |
| 5A | 2000-2400+ | --- |
| 6 | 2000-2400+ | 2400+ |
| 7 | 2000-2400+ | --- |

In general, the higher the donor density, the greater the number of hairs each follicular unit will contain. With low donor density, little scalp laxity or poor hair characteristics, these targets may not be achievable.

We generally do not recommend hair restoration surgery for Class 3 patients unless the hair loss is cosmetically very bothersome, the hair loss pattern seems stable, and the patient has excellent donor reserves. Often these patients have special circumstances, such as career demands, which require transplantation at an early stage. Medications are the best initial treatment, especially with early Class 3 patients.

The number of grafts required to complete the hair transplant process for a given Norwood Class may vary significantly from individual to individual. Nevertheless, it is helpful for someone anticipating surgery to have an idea of the number of follicular units that a typical individual would need for a complete restoration, both with and without crown coverage. (This data was published in Follicular Transplantation: Patient Evaluation and Surgical Planning. Dermatologic Surgery 1997.)

## Total Number of Follicular Units Suggested for a Complete Restoration

| Norwood Class | Follicular Units | Total Units With Crown |
|---|---|---|
| 3 | 900-1500 | --- |
| 3 Vertex | 900-1500 | 1300-2000 |
| 3A | 1400-2200 | --- |
| 4 | 1200-2000 | 1700-3000 |
| 4A | 1800-3600 | --- |
| 5 | 1700-3000 | 2100-4000 |
| 5A | 2000-4400 | --- |
| 6 | 2200-4600 | 3000-5600 |
| 7 | 2200-4800 | 4000-6600 |

A satisfactory restoration does not necessarily mean that complete coverage of the entire bald area has been achieved. Finite donor supplies often limit what can be accomplished, regardless of the hopes of the patient or the abilities of the surgeon. The specific attributes of the patient's hair and the nature of the patient's expectations will both influence the patient's satisfaction with his final results. With an aesthetically planned transplant, many patients can achieve satisfaction with a smaller number of grafts than the above tables suggest. However, for those patients with less than optimal hair characteristics or those with higher expectations, the numbers may be greater.

# 10

## A Hair Transplant at NHI

When you arrive for your hair transplant, the NHI staff will begin by reviewing the surgical process with you. Your NHI physician will review the goals that had been established in prior consultations and will answer any last minute questions. The doctor will take the time to be sure that there are no outstanding issues, areas of confusion or concerns. The surgical consent forms (copies of these forms will be sent to you when you schedule your surgery) will be reviewed and signed, and pre-surgical photographs will be taken.

### Length of the Procedure

Your Follicular Unit Transplant may require many hours of work by a team of professionals. Some of the longest procedures (between 2000-2500+ grafts) may take hours of surgery. During that time, your surgeon and several highly trained technicians and/or nurses will participate in the process. The work must be organized efficiently so that the total length of the procedure for the patient is minimized. On average, a procedure of 1500 grafts would last about 6 hours.

### The Surgical Experience

The procedure may be long, but for the patient the time goes by quickly. You will be given a mild sedative so that you may sleep if desired, or may choose to remain fully awake. Most patients watch television or movies or listen to music for at least part of the time. We try to make your experience enjoyable so that the actual time the surgery takes seems negligible. A relaxed and informal atmosphere is encouraged so that the day goes by quickly and is a pleasurable experience. The patient takes a series of breaks, to the bathroom, to eat lunch, or to just stretch and move around. Patients often tell us that the experience of being the focus of the day's activities is wonderful.

## Anesthesia

After the mild sedative is given orally, you will receive a small series of injections of local anesthetic in the perimeter of the scalp. Any discomfort usually only occurs in the beginning of the anesthetic administration. The actual hair transplant procedure is painless. We also give routine antibiotics during the procedure (but not afterwards).

We use a combination of lidocaine (Xylocaine), which you have probably been given at your dentist, and a longer-acting local anesthetic called Marcaine. Injections around the perimeter of the scalp (called a ring block) will numb the entire scalp, and although this is uncomfortable, a little hand-holding will get you through it just fine. Most of our offices also offer patients nitrous oxide to patients during this time, and it can be of significant help. With this technique, there is no need to apply anesthesia directly into the area that is being transplanted. Once anesthetization is complete, there is generally no pain or discomfort during the remainder of the procedure. If you do require more anesthesia, it will be administered before the first wears off.

We do not perform these operations under general anesthesia (with the patient asleep), as this increases the risks involved in the procedure and is unnecessary. One special note: you will not be permitted to drive yourself home after the procedure, so please arrange to have a family member or friend pick you up.

## The Surgical Team

The hair transplant procedure can be long. After the

removal of the donor strip, the surgical team must work non-stop to dissect the individual hair grafts from the donor strip.

NHI boasts what we consider the most highly skilled of surgical teams in performing microscopically controlled Follicular Unit Transplantation. The team must prepare the grafts according to the surgeon's exact specifications. The preparation and placement of 2,000 or more grafts may take a surgical team hours of intensive, concentrated work. Care must be taken to keep the surgical team free of stress. Just as the patient needs a break, so do team members. At NHI, we focus on the needs of our staff as well as the patient to ensure that the staff is always at peak performance.

## Donor Scalp

The location of the donor strip is carefully selected by your doctor. The hair in this area is clipped short, to a length of approximately 1-mm. This step must be performed with precision. If done properly, the uncut hair will completely cover the donor area when the patient leaves the office.

After the strip of donor scalp is removed, it is temporarily placed into a container with chilled Lactated Ringer's, a solution that closely mimics the body's own natural fluids. The area where the donor strip was removed is sutured closed. This usually leaves a fine scar that heals in a week or two, with the sutures either self-dissolving (the usual case), or being removed. Ideally, the scar will heal well enough to be almost undetectable even when the hair is combed back by a barber or hairdresser.

After the tissue has been harvested, the individual follicular units are meticulously dissected out in their naturally occurring groups, under strict stereomicroscopic control. The grafts are trimmed of extraneous fatty tissue and the hairless intervening skin between the groups is discarded.

The isolation of individual, naturally occurring follicular units and their careful dissection under microscopic control, is an essential part of Follicular Unit Transplantation. If these steps are not performed correctly, the follicles can be injured and their growth impaired. It is important that an experienced surgical team carry out these steps.

## Bleeding

Many people have the impression that hair transplantation is a "bloody procedure." In our hands, it is not. In addition to using very tiny recipient sites, we have developed surgical techniques that greatly minimize the amount of bleeding in all aspects of the procedure. We take many precautions to protect ourselves from all blood-born agents; our patients and staff are routinely tested for HIV and hepatitis for everyone's protection and safety.

## The Surgical Suite

Our surgical team wears masks, surgical gloves, and gowns and only uses instruments that are disposable or sterile. The procedure is performed while you sit in a comfortable, adjustable reclining chair. The surgical rooms are equipped with music, TV, and an assortment of movies.

After the anesthesia is administered, you should feel nothing other than pressure sensations. Many patients have long, friendly conversations with the doctor and assistants during the time it takes to complete the transplant. Occasionally, a patient will speak to friends or conduct business transactions during the surgery on their cell phones. Of course, we would prefer you to take the day off and relax.

The atmosphere in the treatment area makes the patient feel secure and relaxed. Concern and compassion on the part of the doctor and medical staff make a tremendous difference. We all work to make sure that your experience is a pleasant one.

We are proud that New Hair Institute Medical Group, a Professional Corporation (NHI) has been awarded the certificate of accreditation by the Accreditation Association for

Ambulatory Health Care, Inc. The award means that NHI has met nationally recognized standards for quality health care set by the Chicago-based accrediting organization. NHI is the first and only hair transplant clinic in the United States to receive accreditation.

## Making the Recipient Sites

The methods used to create recipient sites for the grafts can add a great deal to the aesthetic look of your transplant. These methods will determine the angle at which the new hair grows as well as distribution and density. Creating recipient sites is a very important part of the procedure, and requires considerable artistic knowledge and surgical skill. It may be the one part of the procedure where your NHI physician is silent as he concentrates on making these sites. Don't be concerned if he isn't chatty during this time.

Your NHI physician is accustomed to working in and around existing hair, so you need not cut your hair short for the procedure. Your existing hair may help to cover any traces of the transplant.

## Placement of New Grafts

The placing of the grafts is the longest and most exacting part of the procedure. During this time, you will be asked to keep your head relatively still. Watching TV, movies or even sleeping will help make the time go quickly. You can takes breaks as needed to eat and use the bathroom.

When placing is complete, photos are taken and post-op instructions are given to you verbally and in writing. A bandage that looks like a tennis headband is placed around your head, and a baseball cap is worn home. No bandages are required on the transplanted area.

## After Your Procedure

The night of the surgery and for a few nights afterwards, you are encouraged to sleep with your head elevated on pillows. You will be given medication to help you sleep if needed. The morning after surgery, you can remove the tennis band and take a shower, gently cleaning the transplanted area with a special shampoo. The follicular unit grafts are made to fit snugly into the recipient sites and will not be dislodged in the shower, if you follow the instructions given to you. After your first shower, no further bandages are required.

If the post-operative instructions are followed carefully, the transplant will be minimally detectable after a few days, and practically undetectable after the first week for most patients. We will give you medication for swelling, but in spite of this, some patients experience swelling of the forehead that settles around the bridge of the nose over the course of the next several days. If this occurs, it is usually gone within a week and should not be a cause for concern.

Frequently, the newly transplanted grafts can be made less noticeable by minor changes in hairstyle and a little bit of hair spray (using the surrounding hair if it is present) to cover the area. Foundation can be used to cover any redness that lasts more than a week. Makeup consultants in large drug stores and department stores can help you choose the appropriate shade and type of makeup. Problems of visibility can also be minimized by altering the appearance of your face. If you do not shave for a while, most people will focus upon your new beard, not on your head. If you have a mustache or a beard, consider shaving it off for the first few weeks and then letting it grow back.

We will call you the morning after your procedure to answer questions and to see if there is anything that you need. You will be given a follow-up appointment approximately two weeks after your procedure. For patients who live far from the office, follow-ups may be handled by phone.

# 11

## What to Expect Following Surgery

After your hair transplant procedure, you will be given written instructions that explain in detail how to care for your scalp until your return visit. Prescriptions for medications may be given at that time (or before the procedure). Most doctors give their patients an analgesic such as Tylenol with codeine. Antibiotics may be prescribed to prevent infection. Some doctors give medication to prevent swelling, although these have limited value. Tranquilizers and sleeping medications are prescribed to help the patient over the first few days of healing.

Immediately following surgery, your grafts are held in place by fibrin (the body's natural glue) produced by a chemical reaction in serum when the graft sites are made. The grafts are loosely held in place for the first 2-3 days and become fully secure at about the eighth day. The hairs that are present in your new grafts usually fall out during the first 2-6 weeks after the procedure (see Growth of New Hair section below). At this time, the patient will usually look just like he did before the transplant. Follicular Unit Transplantation is a relatively minor surgical procedure; most people recover in several days, and many return to work right away. Some discomfort generally exists in the donor site for a few days after the surgery. The discomfort is best managed beyond the first day in most people with Tylenol (with or without codeine). Athletic activities should be restricted for 1-2 weeks. Some limited restrictions apply in the second week. Although we caution patients not to put undue stress on the donor area for several months, normal activity may be resumed 1-2 weeks after the procedure.

There are several different approaches to post-surgical treatment. The patient may leave with no bandage after the surgery or he may be given a small sweatband to keep pressure on the donor area. The recipient area is left open or lightly covered. This enables the transplanted area to be exposed to the air for drying and healing.

Patients often worry about the potential visibility of their new grafts. Scabs that tend to form on the scalp surface should be washed off as they accumulate for the first few days following the surgery. With the very small sites used in Follicular Unit Transplantation, no new crusts will form after the second day. Other than the stubble of transplanted hair and some faint redness, the transplant should not be visible after the first week.

For those individuals who wash their transplanted grafts well, the full extent of the transplant looks and feels (in the days following the procedure) just like a five o'clock shadow. Swelling of the forehead is present in 25% of people between the third and fifth day, but rarely lasts more than one day. Rarely, swelling of the eyelids occurs.

## Sutures

After three years of research, the physicians of the New Hair Institute have switched to a totally absorbable suture for most of our hair transplant procedures. The results of this study, recently published in Dermatologic Surgery concluded "Poliglecaprone 25 (Monocryl) is a very strong synthetic, absorbable, monofilament suture with low tissue reactivity that can be used in hair transplantation to close the donor wound with a single, running cutaneous stitch. If specific surgical techniques are followed, suturing with Monocryl can produce a fine surgical scar superior to metal staples and can result in a more comfortable post-operative experience for the patient."

We are pleased to offer this new suture to our patients. Besides the convenience of not needing to have the suture removed, it is skin colored and is literally invisible, even with the hair relatively short. We still encourage our patients to come by for their 1-week follow-up visit if they live close by, but suture removal is no longer a hassle.

## Growth of New Hair

Growth of new hair appears to be rapid in the first 1-3 weeks, but this usually represents the beginning of the shedding of the hair shafts, which is common as the hair follicles go into a "dormant phase." This phase reflects the shock to the grafts from the transplant process. When the dormant phase occurs, it usually lasts 3-6 months from the time of the transplant before the new hair growth becomes evident. The dormant phase has lasted as long as eight months or longer in a small number of patients. It is during this period that the greatest anxiety occurs. The patient wonders if the hair will ever grow and if the decision to undergo the procedure was a smart one.

In most people, hair growth usually starts within 3-4 months. Growth occurs in cycles, each cycle starting a few days or weeks from the previous cycle. When the hair initially starts growing, the thickness of the shaft is often smaller than normal. This changes as the hair reaches a length of about 1/2 inch. A slow growth process is preferential for most men, because the hair growth is less noticeable. The return of hair reflects a reversal of the balding process, rarely noticed by friends or family as anything out of the ordinary. By 8 months, most people can see the effect of the process, and by 12 months, the growth and bulk will have reached 90% of its total growth. Hair can continue to mature as long as 24 or more months following the transplant procedure. For this reason, patients should not expect to see the preponderance of benefits from the hair transplant process for at least 12 months. Wound healing is relatively fast. The surgical wound in the donor area usually heals within 1-2 weeks, although it may take many months to regain its full strength. In about half of the patients, the transplants on the top and crown of the head are barely visible within the first week. The existing hair can easily hide the donor incision. Those with more persistent redness in the recipient area often have a fair complexion or red hair.

Patients often express doubt or skepticism about the rapidity of the healing process with Follicular Unit Transplantation. Such doubts are most evident in those individuals who received traditional hair transplants because they remember the ugly, obvious wounds on their heads and the impact on their lives after their procedures. For those individuals in particular, it is critical to see and speak with a patient who is one or two weeks post-surgery. Most are more than willing to show prospective patients the results of their work at this early stage.

## Delayed or Reduced Growth

As growth cycles vary widely, some patients may experience significantly delayed growth. This can produce substantial anxiety for these patients. Causes for delayed growth have theoretical explanations (published in the literature as H- or X- factors), however this phenomenon is not well understood and is, fortunately, uncommon. We have seen significant growth between 12-24 months following a hair transplant in a few patients who presented with delayed growth. In the rare case of reduced growth, additional work may be necessary.

## Post-Op Course in Patients Undergoing Follicular Unit Transplantation

The following chart shows the anticipated course for the

average patient undergoing Follicular Unit Transplantation, regardless of the size of the session. This chart is intended to serve as a general guide. It is normal for there to be significant variation between patients and even between sessions in the same patient. Therefore, if you do not follow the course exactly as outlined, do not be concerned.

| TIME POST-OP | TRANSPLANTED AREA | DONOR (Sutured) AREA |
|---|---|---|
| Next Day | Hair is washed thoroughly. Grafts should be clean of blood. | Some soreness, tightness and numbness. |
| 2-3 Days | Scabbing is largely gone. Moderate redness may be present. Some selling may appear on forehead. | Soreness begins to disappear. Some numbness may continue. |
| 1 Week | Redness is minimal to absent. Swelling is usually gone. 1st Post-op Visit. | Soreness generally gone Occasionally some numbness persists. |
| 2 Weeks | Looks and feels like a 4-day -old beard. | Sutures begin to absorb. Discomfort is gone. Numbness is uncommon. |
| 2-8 Weeks | Transplanted hair is shed as the follicles enter a dormant phase. | Knots at the ends of the absorbable sutures fall off. |
| 2-4 Months | Some original hair may be shed in the transplanted area. | Numbness in the in donor area is usually gone. |
| 3-6 Months | Transplanted hair first begins to grow as very fine hair. | |
| 5-10 Months | Some or all of the original hair that was shed begins to grow. | |

| TIME POST-OP | TRANSPLANTED AREA | DONOR (Sutured) AREA |
|---|---|---|
| 8 Months | Hair is groom-able, but trans plant appears thin as hair continues to grow and thicken. Slight changes in the texture of the new hair is occasionally present. | |
| 8-12 Months | Patient is evaluated for a possible second procedure. | |
| 12 Months | 90% of the final appearance of procedure is usually present. | |
| 1-2 Years | There may be additional fullness during the second year. Any change in texture of hair usually returns to normal. | |

# 12

## OTHER SURGICAL HAIR RESTORATION PROCEDURES

This chapter addresses various surgical methods of replacing hair that are still performed, but quickly losing acceptance as viable treatments for most cases of androgenetic alopecia. For the majority of these procedures, the risks to the patient outweigh any potential benefits.

### Occipito-Temporal, Juri, and Other Flaps

"Flap" is the medical term for a piece of skin (in this case on the scalp) that has been cut away from surrounding tissue on three sides. This peninsula of skin remains attached on the fourth side. This side provides the blood supply for the entire flap. Flaps are used to move one piece of skin, such as one that is hair bearing, to a nearby area of the scalp that is bald. One advantage of flaps over "free" skin grafts is that they carry their blood supply with them. Free skin grafts have to develop a blood supply in the area where they are placed. Complex organs, like hair follicles, which might die before they can develop a blood supply, are at less risk when the flap technique of surgery is used. A flap is also one of the few ways that long hair can be redistributed without clipping the donor hairs short.

Designing a scalp flap requires isolating a long artery and the hair-bearing skin that the artery directly supplies. Two long, parallel incisions are made and joined at one end. A strip of skin about 2.5 cm wide is isolated from the surrounding skin except for the attachment at its base (the end of the flap through which the artery enters). After this, the attachments between this strip of skin and the underlying tissue are divided. A recipient site is prepared in the intended area by making an incision and removing the overlying skin. The free end of the flap is then transferred from its original location to the new one. Sewing the skin edges together closes the residual opening in the donor area. Some flap procedures use two flaps, one from each side of the head. Other procedures use a single, long flap from one side and the back of the head.

Flap procedures are major surgery that must be performed in a hospital-level operating room. Some doctors do the operation in two stages. First, they delay the flap by making the peripheral incisions for it, but leaving the flap in place to stimulate the development of an independent arterial blood supply. This creates a barrier of scar surrounding the flap on three sides. The area becomes wholly dependent upon its base artery for its entire blood supply.

Flaps have both advantages and disadvantages. Only physicians who have extensive experience with flaps do these procedures. Patients who are considering flap surgery must be fully informed about the potential complications of the operation and the degree of risks that they take if they choose this option.

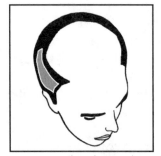 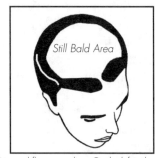

Figure 12–1. These diagrams show a Temporal flap procedure. On the left is the pre-operative view with the shaded area indicating the planned flap. The post-operative view is on the right. The shaded area demonstrates the baldness that remains behind the flap. When the bald area is as wide as shown in this diagram, a second pair of flaps may be done behind the first pair.

*Advantages: Speed*

A flap offers the quickest potential method of putting long, dense hair into a frontal bald area.

*Disadvantages: Necrosis*

The worst possible complication of flap creation is necrosis, the medical term for tissue death. In one study by an experienced plastic surgeon, more than one-third of the flaps sustained some degree of necrosis. The surgeon said that because of the frequency of this problem he would not perform flap surgery any longer. When a flap dies, it leaves a wide, ugly scar in the frontal hairline area of the scalp. This is very difficult to conceal with corrective procedures.

*Disadvantages: Infection*

A possible serious complication of flap surgery is infection, which can cause flap necrosis or permanent hair loss. Areas where the blood supply is temporarily or permanently reduced, such as with a flap procedure, make a rich environment for bacteria to invade and grow.

*Disadvantages: Hair Loss in the Donor Area*

Healthy hair can be lost in the donor area due to infection, trauma or technically poor closure of the surgical wound. Hair lost in this manner leaves a wide, permanent, and unsightly scar in the temple area. Such scars are difficult to hide.

*Disadvantages: Quality and Direction of Hair Growth*

Most flap procedures involve a reversal of scalp position. This means that the hair is forced to grow in the reverse direction of the normal pattern. The reversal of direction gives a distinctly abnormal appearance to one's hair.

In an effort to improve the appearance of a flap, some doctors remove part of the hair from the leading edge of the flap. Other doctors place small grafts of fine hair directly in front of the flap. These techniques attempt to create a zone of finer hair oriented in the proper direction with the goals of hiding the straight line of scar that is often visible in front of the flap and making the flap appear more natural.

### Disadvantages: Broad Frontal Hairline

Because the flap is rotated from the side of the scalp to the front, it creates a broad hairline. It is practically impossible for the surgeon using a flap, to create the soft, tapered look and natural temporal recession that is characteristic of a normal male hairline.

### Disadvantages: Too Much Density in One Area

A flap transfers the full density of the donor area to the frontal hairline. In fact, due to tissue contraction, the flap may even exceed the density of the area from where it originated. As one ages, the frontal hairline normally thins slightly, even in someone who is not balding, so the excessive density of the flap will never look natural. In fact, it will worsen over time as the surrounding area begins to thin. In addition, the flap uses up so much donor hair that there is little left to adequately cover other areas of the scalp.

### Disadvantages: Absence of Hair Behind the Flap

Because the flap can only cover a limited area, the scalp behind the flap remains bald. This area may not be too visible in patients with dense hair, but patients who have sparse hair, or who have highly contrasting hair and skin color, often have difficulty hiding the expanse of bare scalp. Some patients, whose temple hair thins as they age, also have problems with visibility of the bald part of the scalp. These patients typically become extremely self-conscious about their appearance.

There have been cases where men were so desperate that they had the bare scalp tattooed to conceal the baldness. As the tattoo ages, the color fades and the scalp assumes a blue or green color. This results in an undeniably strange appearance. Transplanting hair into this area can improve its general appearance, but the effects of the flap procedure often decrease the number of available grafts and thus can make corrective "repair" work difficult.

*Disadvantages: Excessive Brow*

An excessive brow can occur when loose forehead skin over the eyebrows is pushed down and forward, a movement caused by the flap when it is transposed to the forehead. The patient develops jutting, overhanging eyebrows that give a weird, Neanderthal appearance to the face. This can be corrected by a brow lift operation in which the excess, loose skin in front of the flap is excised. However, proper planning of the procedure by knowledgeable surgeon should prevent this problem.

*Disadvantages: Malposition of the Flaps*

If the flaps are incorrectly placed on one's head, the patient's appearance is truly bizarre.

## Square Grafts

Grafts derived from a linear strip of donor hair can be used as line grafts described below, or can be divided into smaller grafts that are irregular, square, or rectangular. A square graft theoretically contains a few more hairs than a round graft of similar size. A square graft fits into a round or slit site because the graft assumes the shape of the recipient site.

Some surgeons use a square punch to make recipient sites. Proponents of this method point out that, on paper, square shapes can be placed closer together than round ones can. Square shapes do not leave small spaces between them like round ones do. However, because of their square shape, the punches can only be made in large sizes while round punches can be made as small as 1 mm in diameter.

Another problem with square recipient sites concerns the problem of blood supply. A circle is the best shape for allowing the most nutrition to reach the center of the graft. Square grafts have a tendency to become rounded with time and the doughnutting effect from an inadequate blood supply is more pronounced.

## Line Grafts

Some physicians do a procedure in which a 3-4 mm wide linear strip of donor hair is removed, but instead of dividing the strip into miniature grafts, the entire strip (or portions of it) is transplanted into a trench in the recipient area. The line graft procedure presents several problems. First, the equivalent of doughnutting in round grafts increases with line grafts. Second, as the hair in a line graft grows, it appears to be just that: a thin, linear band of hair growing in a straight line that looks extremely unnatural.

## Scalp Reductions

In 1978, two Canadian physician brothers named Blanchard reported a new technique for dealing with baldness in the crown area of the scalp. They excised the bald portion of the scalp and sewed the edges of skin together. The procedure, the "scalp reduction," caught on quickly because at least initially, it seemed to quickly eliminate most of the bald crown. It was also good for the surgeon's practice since the procedure was quick and relatively inexpensive, but locked the patient into further procedures down the line.

Since the original report, several doctors have developed and expanded upon the idea. Several different names have been attached to the procedure: Alopecia Reduction, Galeoplasty, and Male Pattern Reduction (MPR). Once again, the attachment of such names adds unnecessary confusion to the field. We will continue to use the term "scalp reduction" throughout this book.

The procedure entails a minor operation that can be performed in a doctor's office under local anesthesia. The risk of short-term complications is small. The amount of bald scalp that can safely be removed varies greatly from one patient to another, as there are inborn differences in skin and tissue elasticity from one person to another. The natural degree of elasticity of the scalp is graded on a five-point scale. The system is very subjective, and even an experienced doctor can be wrong occasionally.

From the patient's standpoint, the most obvious difference among the many types of scalp reduction is the pattern of the area that is excised. This determines the final shape of the scar. The most common patterns that physicians use are the vertical ellipse and the triangular shape. A few physicians remove crescent shaped areas from the bald part of the scalp directly adjacent to the dense hair.

## Vertical Ellipse Reduction

The vertical ellipse reduction is the most common pattern of excision used to reduce the bald scalp. An ellipse (oval) of bald skin is removed from the center of the bald area running in a direct line from front to back. The procedure is simple, but has one potential problem: a posterior slot deformity. If too much bald area at the very back of the head is removed, it can leave a scar with hair diverging from it on either side. In effect, this looks like the feathered part of an arrow shaft with a series of lines pointing directly at the scar. The scar becomes obvious, and it is almost impossible to hide or correct the deformity.

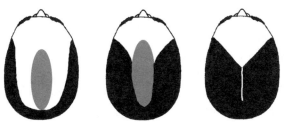

Figure 12–2. A series of three vertical scalp reductions from the pre-operative stage on the left to the final result on the right. The shaded area represents the planned reduction.

French physician, Dr. Patrick Frechet, has developed a clever procedure to conceal a posterior slot deformity. The procedure creates pedicles of skin that are rotated into the excised area. Hair from these pedicles break up the abnormal "slot" by introducing still another direction of hair growth. This confuses the eye, thereby lessening the effect of the deformity.

## Triangular "Mercedes Star" Reduction

The triangular pattern of excision for a scalp reduction has several advantages. It removes the largest portion of bald scalp from the center of the baldest area. It also elevates the lower edge of the bald area and raises it toward the top of the crown area. It is sometimes called the "Mercedes Star" procedure because its final shape resembles the shape of the Mercedes Benz symbol. However, this means that the patient is branded with a "Mercedes Star" for life. With an extensive degree of reduction, slot deformities occur with this procedure as well, but they are usually minimal and correctable.

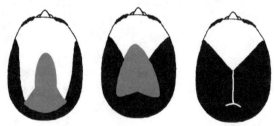

Figure 12–3. A series of three triangular scalp reductions from the pre-operative stage on the left to the final result on the right. The shaded area represents the planned reduction.

## Multi-Z Reduction

The multi-z reduction is a variant of the vertical ellipse or triangular reduction procedure. It is usually reserved for the last of a series of scalp reduction procedures. Instead of a straight line, the two sides of the incision are cut in a pattern of matching "saw teeth" so that they mesh. Longitudinal scars contract along their long axis making the scar more prominent. By breaking up a single long scar into a series of shorter ones, the contraction of a long scar is avoided. With this technique, a more cosmetically pleasing result is obtained; dense hair on either side of the incision often hides the scar, so that further procedures or grafts may not be needed. This procedure also reduces the possibility of creating a slot deformity.

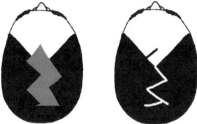

Figure 12–4. A Multi-Z scalp reduction from the pre-operative stage on the left to the final result on the right. The shaded area represents the planned reduction.

Some doctors use a series of lateral excisions at the back and sides of the head to remove an area of baldness that is limited to the back part of the crown. Because the scar is at least partly hidden by the dense hair next to it, a lateral scalp reduction may be much more cosmetically pleasing than a vertical or triangular one. The latter two procedures leave a scar in the center of the baldest area. A scar in the center of a relatively bare area will be much more noticeable than one that is next to dense hair.

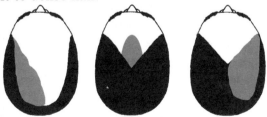

Figure 12–5. A series of three semilunar scalp reductions from the pre-operative stage on the left to the penultimate stage on the right. The shaded area represents the area of planned reduction.

## Hair Lift

A hair lift is a more radical type of scalp reduction. In the more common types of scalp reductions described above, the scalp skin is dissected or loosened down to a level just above the major blood vessels of the scalp. In a hair lift, the dissection or loosening is to a level below the major blood vessels of the scalp. To avoid damage to these blood vessels, the nerves are deliberately cut and tied. This allows removal of a larger area of bald skin in a single operation instead of doing a series of smaller ones, but it often leaves the head permanently numb. These patients no longer enjoy the feeling of someone massaging their heads or running a comb through their scalps. Unlike other scalp reductions, this major surgical procedure must be performed under general anesthesia and in a hospital-level surgical setting. It also has the disadvantage of leaving visible scars around the ears. A side effect of this procedure is that additional hair may be lost due to the surgical stress; however, this hair loss is usually temporary. In addition, the donor supply is often significantly depleted, severely limiting any benefit from possible future hair transplant procedures.

## Scalp Expansion and Scalp Extension

Scalp expanders are silicone balloons inserted into pockets created between the under surface of the scalp and the skull. After allowing several weeks for the scalp incisions to heal, the balloons are gradually inflated with a series of injections of salt solution. The inflated balloons cause the head to swell to two or three times its normal size. The redundant skin that results is then excised. Scalp expanders are very useful in cases where traumatic loss of hair has occurred, especially in children or in burn patients, however they are not usually used for patients with male pattern hair loss.

With scalp extensions, an internal device is used to pull hair-bearing areas closer together without the deformity of the balloon expanders. This technique, developed by Dr. Patrick Frechet, a set of springs is placed inside the scalp. These springs stretch the scalp and produce overlapping scalp tissue.

The excess skin is removed once it reaches it maximum stretch. The spring-like device is placed inside the scalp and removed some weeks or months later along with the excess skin.

*Advantages of Scalp Reductions*

The one significant advantage to scalp reductions is that in less than one hour, the balding area in the crown often can be reduced by 3-4 cm in width and 12 cm in length. The benefits are immediate. Occasionally, we see a patient with a bald spot that is 5-6 cm wide and who has hyper-elastic skin. In these patients, it may be possible to remove the entire bald area in the crown in a single 30-minute procedure.

*Disadvantages: Stretchback*

Many physicians have begun to question the advisability of doing scalp reductions. They have cited the occurrence of "stretchback" as a reason not to do the procedure. Stretchback is a phenomenon in which the stretched part of the dense hair area widens out. The advantage gained by the scalp reduction is partially or totally lost. Some of the doctors who criticize scalp reduction say that they see stretchback in the first few weeks after the procedure. Other doctors report that they do not see significant stretchback.

*Disadvantages: Sterility*

Scalp reductions should be performed under more sterile conditions than are required for other types of hair restoration. Some doctors perform the procedure under the same clean standard that is used for hair transplants, but this is not enough to prevent complications. Nevertheless, scalp reductions are generally categorized as minor surgery and total antisepsis is not required.

*Disadvantages: Shock Hair Loss*

Sometimes hair on both sides of the incision is temporarily lost for a distance of 1-2 cm. The cause of this phenomenon is not clear. Hair that is lost because of surgical shock usually re-grows in three to four months, but there may not be complete re-growth.

### Disadvantages: Accelerated Hair Loss

Accelerated hair loss is more common with scalp reductions than most surgeons care to admit. The natural course of hair loss, which may normally take years, is accelerated, and the loss occurs in weeks or months. The process usually begins within 12 months of the scalp reduction. Hair starts falling out in significant quantities and may never return. The scars that are usually hidden in the corrected area may eventually become visible.

### Disadvantages: Thinning of the Scalp

The scalp tissue thins because of the stretching of the skin from the reduction. Some people develop chronic wounds in the surgical scars of the scalp reduction that recur with some frequency. This is usually the result of closing the reduction under too much tension, and can be corrected with a scar revision procedure.

### Disadvantages: Scarring

Noticeable scars are frequent side effects of scalp reductions.

### Disadvantages: Direction of Hair Growth

With a scalp reduction, hair grows away from the center of the head as the sides are advanced to the center. This creates an unnatural appearance and highlights the balding area and any scars that occur.

As scalp reductions are considered a minor surgical procedure, the chances of complications are low. The risks associated with scalp reductions are as follows.

### Risks: Infection

Although there is a theoretical risk of severe, widespread

infection with scalp reductions, this phenomenon has not been reported. Minor, localized infections occur, but such infections are seen in fewer than 1% of patients who have this procedure.

*Risks: Posterior Slot Deformity*

The complication of posterior slot deformity is frequently seen in patients who have had multiple midline scalp reductions. As more bald area at the very back of the head is removed, a scar is created with hair diverging from it on either side. As discussed under the vertical ellipse reduction, a slot deformity can create an effect similar to the feathered part of an arrow shaft, with a series of lines pointing directly at the scar. It makes the scar obvious, and almost impossible to hide.

*Risks: Hemorrhage*

Bleeding can occur during any surgical procedure. Because of the relatively small size of the blood vessels involved in this operation, and because of their relative accessibility, hemorrhaging during a scalp reduction procedure is easily controlled. Delayed hemorrhage can occur if the patient does any activity that suddenly raises his blood pressure to very high levels, such as heavy weight lifting. Because the blood vessels are superficial, and because the skull underlies them, simple, direct pressure will control any postoperative bleeding until medical help arrives.

*Risks: Hematoma Formation*

A hematoma is a blood clot within the tissues of the body. A hematoma forms in a scalp reduction when a blood vessel begins to bleed after the incision is closed. Like a hemorrhage, the formation of a hematoma may follow unusual physical exertion. If the hematoma is enlarging, active bleeding is occurring, and direct pressure should be applied just below its lowest point, i.e. the area closest to the neck. Immediate medical attention is needed.

## Risks: Suture Reaction

When a scalp reduction is performed, the deeper layers below the skin must be sutured together. An absorbable suture is used for this purpose. On rare occasions, the body rejects this suture material causing pain and swelling, and occasionally the body tries to expel the suture. If the body tries to expel the suture material, holes will appear in the scalp with what is called a "suture sinus." This complication is treated by removing the deep sutures with a minor surgical procedure or just waiting out the process and allowing the body to dissolve the suture material over months.

## A General Assessment of Scalp Reductions

Scalp reductions became popular at a time when the hair restoration alternatives were large plugs and flaps. In the modern era of hair restoration surgery, where transplantations of large numbers of follicular unit grafts are possible, any potential advantage of this procedure is far more limited. There has been some recent interest in overcoming some of the technical problems of scalp reduction surgery, such as reducing stretch back, avoiding mid-line scars with different patterns of reductions, and shortening the total time to achieve a desired result. The problems, however, are more than technical.

A balding patient's appearance is most naturally improved by placing hair in the most important cosmetic areas, the hairline and the front part of the scalp, as these provide a natural frame to the face. Since the crown is generally the least cosmetically important of the balding areas (but potentially the largest), crown coverage should not be a first priority. It should be addressed after the more aesthetically important areas have been satisfactorily transplanted. If treated sooner, there must be sufficient donor reserves to handle any future loss, or the surgeon must be certain that the front has little risk of baldness.

The potential cosmetic improvement is ultimately limited

by a finite donor supply. This, in turn, is strictly dependent upon donor density and scalp laxity. Scalp reductions have the undesirable consequence of decreasing the effective amount of hair that can be moved to the cosmetically critical front and top of the scalp by simultaneously decreasing the donor density and scalp laxity.

As a result of the scalp reduction, a larger donor area must be harvested to yield the same amount of hair. This quantity of hair now becomes more difficult to remove due to a tighter scalp, especially after multiple reductions. When the strip is removed, some of the hair must then be placed back in the crown to cover the scar produced by the reduction. It has been explained by proponents of the operation that a scalp reduction conserves hair by decreasing the size of the bald crown, but in reality, the hair that is used to cover the crown will not be available for the front and top. The reduction, by moving the relatively high density of the back and sides upward is, in actuality, committing large amounts of hair to the back of the scalp.

Because the aesthetically critical front portion of the scalp is significantly smaller in size than the back, the transplantation of extensive numbers of very small grafts can almost always produce satisfactory coverage of the front and the top of the scalp. For patients with limited donor reserves, there is often not enough hair to cover the entire scalp. It is in the best interest of these patients to provide very light coverage to the crown, or leave it bare. However, once the crown is altered by a scalp reduction, the situation changes dramatically. Hair must now be placed in the crown to cover the scar caused by the reduction itself. The scalp reduction scar eliminates the option of leaving the crown untreated. In a patient who becomes extensively bald, this can be a major problem.

In patients who might traditionally be considered ideal candidates for a reduction, such as those with a loose scalp, limited balding, and a bare crown that is cosmetically very both-

ersome, crown coverage can easily be accomplished with follicular unit transplantation by creating a delicate swirl in the
center with one, two, and three hair units spiraling outward.
The transplanted swirl will now provide for natural, permanent coverage if the bald area expands, minimizing the need
for further surgery. Furthermore, in patients with moderate
donor density, only a conservative amount of hair is committed to the crown. When greater donor density permits, fuller
crown coverage can be accomplished. In both instances, the
original direction of hair is maintained, crown balding can
progress in its natural radial pattern, and there is no scar.

The scalp reduction hampers the ability to reduplicate the
delicate swirl of hair that normally defines the crown and can
create future problems. Since the scalp reduction scar is linear or geometric, the hair used to cover it will follow the same
pattern. Eventually, as the balding progresses, the hair will
recede from the area, leaving an isolated patch of hair in the
same unnatural pattern as the scar it originally served to
cover. The crown will then demand more hair to follow this
new expanding cosmetic problem. After a reduction, the
scarred skin, the irregular balding pattern, and the abnormal
direction of hair may preclude the crown from ever looking
normal. This is a significant price to pay for a short-term cosmetic improvement in the back of one's scalp.

# 13

## HAIR SYSTEMS

In this chapter, we will look at synthetic methods of simulating the look of a normal head of hair. Most often, these are hairpieces, toupees, wigs, or just "pieces." The discussion below is true for all hairpieces.

Hairpieces start with a section of netting, called the foundation. The netting is cut and molded to approximate the size and shape of the bald scalp area. The highest quality and most natural-looking hairpieces are custom-made and may cost thousands of dollars. They are made of high quality human hair, carefully matched to the original hair of the client. The hairs, singly or in very tiny bunches, are skillfully tied around the threads of the foundation netting and knotted so that they lay in directions that follow the pattern of natural hair growth. All wigs are fragile and must be returned regularly to the maker for cleaning and upkeep; they usually last only a few years. Sun, salt water, the chlorine in swimming pools, and harsh shampoos all shorten the life of a hairpiece. Most clients have two of them: one is in use while the other is in the shop.

Considering manufacture, upkeep, and replacement, the expense of wigs is significant, and the client must expect continued expense throughout his life. The hairs of less expensive wigs may be made of artificial fibers, animal hair, or human hair, but human hair has the most natural appearance and behavior. The less expensive and most common wigs are made from Asian hair that is dyed or bleached to approximate Caucasian coloring. The texture is never convincing, and although Asian hair is very strong, the bleaching and toning processes make it brittle and dry so that the strands break easily. For this reason, cheap hairpieces are less durable and begin to look fuzzy very quickly; they must be replaced at frequent intervals.

Hairpieces are the most popular and widely used method of hair replacement. For men whose baldness is very extensive, a hairpiece may be the only alternative to hair transplantation or shaving the scalp. The cost and the final appearance of a hairpiece varies with the materials used and the expertise of the maker.

The major advantages of wearing a hairpiece are the initial cost and convenience. The change is immediate and there is usually no medical procedure involved. A well-made hairpiece should need adjustment about as often as an average, non-bald man needs to have a haircut.

There are many long-term disadvantages to hairpieces: lack of durability, cleaning, the need for duplicates, unnatural frontal hairlines, and accelerated hair loss of the hair covered by the hairpiece.

## Durability

Human hair is fragile. Living hair is always breaking off, and the ends may tend to split. The hair in a hairpiece cannot replace itself as growing hair does. One must replace the hairpiece at intervals that depend upon the quality of the hairpiece and the client's concern for his or her appearance.

## Cleaning

Some types of hairpieces are easy for the client to remove and replace. This allows more frequent scalp cleansing than with permanently attached hairpieces. The client must choose between convenience and security; both have advantages and drawbacks. Shampooing cannot remove skin cells, skin oils, shed hair, and other debris that accumulates between the netting and the scalp with a permanent hairpiece. These kinds of hairpieces must be removed from time to time to clean the piece and the underlying hair and scalp.

## Duplicates

Many clients have a second hairpiece made to wear while the first is being cleaned and perhaps re-styled. The initial expense of this option is justified by the increased lifespan of both pieces.

## Frontal Hairline

Unless the client has natural hair remaining in his frontal hairline, the border of the hairpiece may be highly visible, tending to separate from the scalp and leaving a visible line. Hiding this space can be the most difficult challenge of the wigmaker's art. However, an experienced craftsperson can accomplish this, and the results can be excellent.

## Accelerated Hair Loss

Some hairpieces have the effect of accelerating hair loss. This may be caused by some of the methods of attachment or the physical or psychological stress induced by the hairpiece. One example is seen with a pair of identical twins. In identical twins, hair loss is virtually identical, but in this case, it was not. One twin used a hairpiece and experienced greater hair loss than his sibling who did not use a hairpiece.

## Methods of Attachment:

The greatest worry for any person who wears a hairpiece is that it will unpredictably come off and be extremely embarrassing. Wig makers have put much effort into devising methods to attach the pieces securely. Each solution has advantages and disadvantages.

### Tape

Tape with adhesive on both sides is one of the simplest

methods of attaching a hairpiece. Tape, however, can leave a sticky residue of adhesive on both the skin and the net foundation of the hairpiece. In addition, tape tends to become unglued when the hair is pulled or when the wearer sweats. This type of attachment is especially unsuitable for people who like to exercise in hot, sunny weather. Swimming and diving also tend to loosen the attachment of taped-on hairpieces.

## Clips and Snaps

Metal clips or snaps can be sewn to the foundation netting. Clips fasten directly to one's natural hair. Snaps are tied or sewn to the netting and to the client's hair. Snaps must be relocated as the hair grows out and the attachment loosens. These methods of fixation are secure, and they have the advantage that the hairpiece can easily be removed so the client can cleanse his scalp. Metal clips are ideal for affixing a hairpiece during the transition phase when a client wants to use a hairpiece to cover his baldness while the new hair of a hair transplant is growing out.

## Weaves

In this method, strands of the client's own hair are pulled through the openings in the foundation mesh of a hairpiece. The client's hair is then woven through the hairpiece foundation to secure it. This method fixes the hairpiece very securely and naturally because of its many points of attachment. Weaves, however do require adjustment as the hair grows to keep the hairpiece closely applied to the client's scalp. In addition, when touched, hair with a weave feels very strange. Weaves often pull on existing hair weakened by the balding process. The constant pull may cause localized, premature hair loss. This mechanism is called traction alopecia.

## Tunnel Grafts

In this technique, tunnels of skin are created in the skin of the client's scalp. These tunnels are made from the client's own skin with skin grafts taken from another area of the body. Usually, three tunnels are made, one in the front and two in the back. Plastic or nylon hooks are sewn to the hairpiece. When the hooks are inserted into the tunnels, the attachment is quite secure, and the hairpiece can easily be removed and replaced by the client without a visit to the wigmaker's salon. The obvious disadvantage of this procedure is that minor surgery is required to create the tunnels. If the tunnels are removed later, permanent scars remain in the scalp. Hair transplants can easily cover the scars on the back of the head left by the tunnels; however, the scar in front may be difficult to conceal.

## No No's

Two procedures involving hairpieces have been set aside for special attention because of the risks and serious consequences involved: sew-ons and the implantation of artificial fibers. These last two methods are mentioned only as a warning against their use. The damage of a scarred scalp is very difficult to hide or cover. We have seen patients seriously deformed by these techniques and advise against them.

## Sew-Ons

One practice is to sew the hairpiece directly onto the client's scalp with an encircling, permanent surgical suture attaching the hairpiece to the scalp. This procedure is illegal in the United States. Unfortunately, in at least one state (New Jersey) some companies have been able to practice their witchcraft for years despite attempts by the New Jersey attorney general to put an end to this activity.

Skin is a more complex organ than most people realize. One of the skin's essential functions is to prevent bacteria and viruses in the environment from entering the bloodstream and the vital organs. When a suture is placed through the skin, it leaves a small hole that allows bacteria, to migrate into the fatty tissue under the skin. This can easily result in infection and abscesses. Many sutures incite enough of an allergic reaction to cause the suture to be rejected and extruded by the skin. Surgical sutures left in the skin for too long cut through the skin and may need replacement. This process is hastened when any traction is applied to the sutures. Though there are a few types of sutures that may remain within the skin for a very long time without causing any problem, most are rejected. Between the sutures, the scars that they cause, and the recurrent infections, a wall of scar tissue gradually builds up in a complete circle around the periphery of the scalp. This encircling wall of scar eventually causes almost total blockage of any blood supply to the central portion of the scalp, as its blood supply comes upward from the surrounding part of the head. A thin, parchment-like layer of scar tissue replaces the skin in the center of the scalp. Any permanent hair that was present in the area surrounded by the suture is also destroyed. The damage is permanent.

## Artificial Fibers

The manufacturer of a synthetic polymer known as "NIDO" claims that the product looks and feels like human hair. This material comes in small bundles of fibers, which are implanted directly into the scalp. It is most widely used in Japan and is available in other countries, but not in the United States. Be careful before you consider this option, as its short- and long-term safety is in question. These artificial fibers are associated with many problems:

| | |
|---|---|
| **Cost** | Usually $2-$3 per hair fiber. |
| **Extrusion** | 15%-25% of the fibers are pushed out of the scalp each year. |
| **Breakage** | The artificial fibers are brittle, and tend to break off at the skin level. |
| **Infection** | Many patients develop chronic infections at the sites of the implants. It is almost impossible to |

treat this type of infection without removing the foreign material.

**Sebum Plugs**   Plugs of fatty material build up at the bases of the fibers and have to be specially cleansed.

**Maintenance**   Every few weeks, the patient has to be treated for infection and have the sebum plugs removed. Over time, this is expensive and probably painful.

**Replacement**   At least once a year, lost and broken fibers have to be replaced.

**Look**   The nylon fibers have a shinier appearance than natural hair.

**Feel**   The artificial fibers have an artificial, stiff texture that does not feel like real hair.

**Styling**   Combing the synthetic fibers is difficult because traction can break them or pull them out.

**Heat**   Use of a hair dryer will cause the fibers to frizz, and damage to the fibers above the skin level is permanent.

**Inflammation**   Infection caused by fiber implants may cause premature loss of natural hair follicles adjacent to the artificial fibers. Over time, inflammation may destroy the scalp to the extent that further hair transplants of any kind are difficult or impossible.

*[The authors are indebted to Dr. Richard Shiell of Melbourne, Australia, for the description of the problems seen with the use of "NIDO" fibers. Because this material is not used in the U.S., we have seen only a few patients who have had these implants, and we have never seen a patient with the material still in place. All of the patients we have seen have had damage from this material. Dr. Shiell has seen patients who still have the material in place.]*

# 15

## DOING YOUR HOMEWORK

A proper assessment of both the quality and quantity of hair required for reconstruction requires a thorough understanding of the amount and cost of work required to achieve a defined result. A doctor must ascertain whether the patient's intended budget can realistically accommodate his needs and expectations. Prospective patients should expect the physician to define, in writing, the expectations and the cost of the work. Ideally, the doctor should describe his impression of the goals that were defined during the consultation and what the proposed treatment is intended to accomplish for that patient. The doctor should also give a prospective patient the opportunity to see and speak with others who have had the procedures being offered. This benefits both parties: it ensures that the patient's expectations are realistic and the patient is able to make an informed decision.

The well being of the patient depends upon the physician's integrity. The physician must educate and inform the prospective patient about the realities of the services being offered. The patient should be informed of all available options, what he will experience, what the visual effect will be, and how much it will cost. The patient should have time to carefully consider the information and have all questions answered. The patient should not rush to schedule the procedure, but rather take deliberate steps to delay the decision until the analysis is complete. A good doctor maintains careful post-operative follow-up of his patients and ensures they return for observation. Matching the patient's results with his or her expectations is an important part of the physician's educational obligation to the patient. An ongoing assessment of the patient's results over time is part of the service the transplant patient should expect to receive.

Many hair restoration physicians produce brochures and/or videos to give prospective patients a clear idea of what the procedure entails, or (less helpfully) to sell them on having surgery. NHI has produced an informative video and extensive collection of printed material, all of which are provided to prospective patients before their initial consultations. This ensures that the patient is educated and prepared to ask questions before meeting with the doctor. The consultation visit is more valuable when the patient is more informed and can ask better questions.

When you decide that you may be interested in surgical hair restoration, it is a sound idea to plan to spend a specific block of time doing research. Many patients take six months to one year to study the procedures available, meet with different doctors and patients, and then make informed decisions to go forward with surgery or not. Planning to take some time in research will help you avoid the pitfalls of becoming an uninformed patient or being "sold" on a procedure before you are ready.

## The Consultation

The initial interviewer should provide you with basic information about the hair transplant procedure. You should fill out a basic medical history form to determine your candidacy for having a surgical procedure. Some assessment of your hair loss may be done at this time, but no one except a physician or a specially qualified nurse practitioner may legally perform a physical examination and render an opinion.

A more knowledgeable interviewer may try to determine if your expectations are realistic. Some salespersons or patient educators work independently in "consultation offices" that are without a physician. Be sure that you are not given the impression that the salesperson is a physician. Also make certain that salespeople do not recommend the type of surgical procedure to be used, the number of procedures or the approximate cost of your restoration without input from a doctor. In some offices, the initial interview is done by a person who is introduced as a "Medical Associate," but that person may be a salesman focused on determining how much money you have and on selling you the procedure. Do not to discuss your financial status before meeting with the doctor.

When a physician is available in the office, the educator or salesman should call the doctor in to examine your scalp, determine the amount of donor hair you have, address your worst-case balding pattern, and then discuss your surgical options. At this stage, the doctor can then review costs with you. Other physicians do the entire consultation themselves: educating the patient, taking a history, doing the physical examination, discussing the options, and reviewing cost.

## See It Before You Believe It!

Ask to meet patients of the medical group you are considering. Be sure that you meet with someone who has a transplant technique similar to the one you might have. Meeting and talking with patients will enhance your confidence in your selection of a doctor. Talk to the doctors about their experience. Look closely at the quality of the doctor's work; by seeing the results of the process you will know whether the work meets your standards. Do not go forward with any procedure until you have had all your questions answered. This is an all-too-often shady business, so there is there is no substitute for good research. Take the time to do your homework. The rewards of a good hair transplant are well worth your effort, time, and research.

NHI often uses actual patients to educate prospective candidates. People who have undergone surgery can relate their motivations for having surgery and their experiences, as well as show their results.

# 16

## ESTABLISH REALISTIC GOALS AND EXPECTATIONS

Realistic expectations are essential to the success of hair transplantation; setting them is the responsibility of both doctor and patient. The doctor must provide each patient with enough information to make an informed decision. This is the doctor's legal obligation. Every hair follicle lost because of genetic balding (androgenic alopecia) is lost forever. If you compare a head of hair to an apple, as the balding process progresses, parts of the apple are being lost. In cases of advanced baldness (a person with a Norwood Class 7 baldness pattern), such a person has lost up to 75% of the apple and as such, he should not reasonably expect to get a full head of hair back. It would be impossible for anyone to make 25% of an apple look like 100% of an apple. However, if 20% of the apple was lost, a skilled person could reconstruct the apple so that the missing 20% could be disguised. The goal of a hair restoration procedure is to make a patient appear to have more hair than he actually has. This is where the art form must be balanced against the technical skills of the surgeon. The combination of art and technique cannot overcome limitations in the quality or quantity of the supply of hair. Generally, the more hair lost, the less full the appearance of the restored hair. All hair restoration procedures, including hair transplantation, actually move hair from one place on the head to another. New hair is not created, but redistributed from the back and sides of the head (where there is an abundant supply) to areas where there is little or none. No surgical procedures create new hair. Scalp reductions do not preserve hair for use in transplants, as some physicians claim, for the same wreath of permanent hair is stretched to cover a wider area in the crown, thereby thinning it. Flaps move large areas of hair from the wreath of permanent hair, leaving significant scarring and distortion of scalp anatomy in the process. Traditional large 4 mm hair transplant grafts, transfer plugs of hair into bald areas, creating patches of hairy skin and thus create the doll's head look, so commonly associated with hair transplants.

In modern hair transplantation, very small naturally growing groups of hair follicles are moved. These follicular grafts are less noticeable than larger grafts and are often indistinguishable from the natural groups of hair growing in adjacent areas of the scalp. The grafts are placed into a pinhole that may leave no discernible scar. The density of the transplanted hair in its new location cannot equal the density of the hair that was originally in that location. In thinning areas, transplanted hair can significantly increase the apparent density by adding hair follicles or groups of hairs and mixing these with existing hair. The key is to add density inconspicuously. The hair in the new location must appear as full and natural as possible.

Unless a very bald man has a high hair density and a loose scalp, there is not enough hair to cover the entire head. A very thin head of hair, a very conservative, high hairline, and/or deliberately leaving the crown area un-grafted or very thin, may be the only available options; this must be understood when a patient makes the decision to have surgery. This is particularly true if the patient's hair density is below average. In patients with extensive hair loss and low-density of donor hair, there is no way that transplantation can achieve a full head of hair. Special artistic techniques, however, can exploit what hair remains. Many of these individuals will be satisfied with a high hairline that does not have a distinct edge. This produces a natural but well-framed thin look. High contrast hair-to-skin color combinations make more advanced hair loss harder to restore.

Both the patient and the doctor bring their own expectations to the process. For the patient, there is no substitute for doing proper research into the subject. Patients must accept the responsibility for their actions and choices if they fail to do the necessary research prior to having surgery. Anyone contemplating such services can only protect himself by educating himself.

A patient's education should include reading general material on the subject that has been produced by the doctor being considered for the transplant service. A review of this material can reveal a great deal about the particular medical group; it will also tell you whether the doctor wants educated patients.

An educated consumer should learn to recognize marketing gimmicks and how such gimmicks can be used to set false expectations in selling hair transplants. Beware of a one-sided, very positive interview. Educating prospective patients and giving them the information necessary, including negative information, to make these very important decisions with confidence is the purpose of the interview with the doctor.

## Coverage Goals

The doctor must discuss your hopes and expectations in light of the physical realities and financial constraints of your particular case. NHI affiliated physicians will work with you to develop realistic goals that are possible to achieve. It is impossible to determine exactly how many procedures it will take to accomplish the coverage you may want. Many people change their goals as their perspective changes with more hair. What we call "hair greed" often reflects a high satisfaction with the initial hair transplant and must be calculated into your decision-making formula.

## Hairline Design

The doctor should sketch a hairline on your head and photograph you so that you can give your insights on a hairline location that meets your needs, your family and ethnic background, and your budget. The choice of hairline (how high, how flat, etc.) is very personal and depends on your head, facial shape, ethnicity, family characteristics, hair reserves, and personal goals. We generally discourage hairlines that do not reflect a maturing pattern because we fully expect that every one of our patients will live to be old.

## Designing the Distribution of Your Hair

In general, we will transplant your hair in a natural distribution, (the way it naturally grows), so you may groom it as you choose. This is realistic in individuals who have above average hair densities and/or more than enough hair to gain the desired coverage for the area being covered. In individuals with low-density hair or an extensive balding area, weighting the hair to one side or the other may produce better coverage from the hair that can be safely harvested. In some instances where a patient has had previous transplants that were improperly distributed, and the patient has a limited donor supply, we may choose to distribute the repair transplants in a way that will most effectively camouflage the existing transplants.

## Styling Tricks and Adjuncts

A patient can make his hair appear thicker by using various mousses, gels and wetting agents. In addition, having a permanent can make straight hair wavy. A good hair stylist can make what we might consider poor hair characteristics look like better hair characteristics. In addition, scalp-coloring agents, which come in many product forms, can color the scalp to reduce high contrast between skin and hair color. By combining styling products with the talents of a good stylist and a skilled hair transplant surgeon, many individuals can achieve fuller results than with hair transplantation alone. This is particularly important for individuals who have depleted their donor supplies by having surgery that used older techniques.

## Financial Planning with Your Budget

Your financial situation will determine how many grafts or how much work you can afford. You should not rush into the transplant process unless you can afford to follow-up with enough work to leave you with a normal appearance. To facilitate this, NHI offers various treatment plans and financing programs to patients who qualify. In these situations, the goals of the patient must be based on economics. Often, a patient is inclined to do only the work he feels he can afford rather than to follow the recommended treatment plan. Patients should clearly understand the aesthetic consequences of purchasing less than the recommended number of grafts. The doctor should be inflexible when it comes to creating a "work in progress" that will lead to an unhappy outcome. Hair restoration surgery is elective surgery and because it is elective, there is plenty of time to think about it thoroughly before commencing the process. In our experience, a major cause for patient dissatisfaction is associated with moving less hair than was recommended. Often, we advise patients to wait until financial resources can be balanced with an appropriate procedure that is designed to meet reasonable goals. The rate of hair loss must also be taken into account, particularly in young men with early, rapid onset balding or thinning.

## Financial Planning for the Progressive Nature of Hair Loss

Given the large number of grafts we routinely place in a single session at NHI, a patient may find that all the work he or she will ever require is accomplished in a single session. However, the patient's balding pattern often dictates the necessity of additional procedures. This is the case when the restoration involves following a receding hairline, particularly in a young patient just starting on his balding pattern. After the initial procedure, the patient is committed to additional procedures as his hairline recedes; the patient must clearly understand the financial commitment he is entering into before having his first surgery. Each hair loss patient has a natural stopping point. Completing the restoration process to this point will allow the patient to have an aesthetically acceptable result. Some individuals can stop after one procedure and some cannot. It is imperative that an individual recognize the category he is in before commencing his hair restoration program.

## Patients with Previous Hair Restoration Surgeries

Unfortunately, more than 1 million men started the hair transplant process with pencil-size grafts. This produced the well-known cornrow or doll's head look that characterizes the early hair restoration era. In addition, these older procedures were frequently wasteful of hair and produced significant scarring around the sides and back of the head. These early techniques produced cosmetic deformities that may    possibly be repaired or corrected with Follicular Unit Transplantation.

1. Hair Restoration History: Your history allows your physician to estimate the required work and the availability of donor hair. The following information is collected:
   • Number and type of procedures, names of physicians, and dates,
   • Condition of donor area and donor area scars from pre vious surgeries, and
   • Description of current hair systems.
2. Satisfaction and Need for Camouflage: The patient (working closely with the physician) will determine his priorities for additional work. Often focusing on making the hairline look more natural by hiding or removing plugs or scars.
3. Characterization of Donor Area: This critical assessment is needed to determine how much movable hair is left in the donor area. This will determine how much total additional work can be done and the number of grafts that may be

attempted in each additional procedure.

4. Status of the Recipient Areas: Each patient should create a list of the goals to be addressed. As the donor supply is often limited, this list will be the basis of a new Master Plan for the repair. Many times, the list may be more extensive than the donor supply can support. Compromises may be necessary, because once the donor supply is fully exploited, further hair restoration procedures will not be possible. This list must not only to itemize the hair coverage issues, but also problems such as cobblestoning, scarring and plugginess. All of the above information will be used to create a unique plan for each patient.

## Realities of Rebuilding Your Hairline

Regaining the hair density of your youth is not a realistic goal. Although some doctors may claim that high hair density can be achieved without a "pluggy" appearance, such claims are misleading. There number of hairs that can be redistributed to cover your balding areas is finite.

In addition to the problems inherent in redistributing a limited amount of hair, there are also limitations on how close together transplanted hair can be  placed. A relatively thick hairline can give the illusion of more hair and fullness, but achieving this natural appearance is not easy.  Auto-transplantation is the science of moving an organ or tissue from one part of the body to another part. Hair follicles constitute an organ that includes the vital support structures needed for the hair to live and grow.

Figure 16–1. Fresh hair grafts positioned in the scalp immediately after 1 session.

123

Because of the need to preserve the sustaining organ during the hair transplant procedure; the physician must extract a safe amount of tissue surrounding the follicle. This extra tissue limits how closely hair can be packed together. Though it may be difficult to mimic nature's density, certain techniques allow the packing of hair to create a natural appearance. In addition to the problems associated with transplanting follicles containing extra tissue, the volume of the scalp also affects the ability to densely pack hair grafts. By placing follicles into the holes placed in the scalp, there is an increase in mass in the area of transplant. If the holes are too close, the insertion of grafts in one section will force grafts out of adjacent sections.

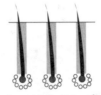

Figure 16–2. Hair grafts in the scalp shown after healing process has occurred. Excess transplanted tissue has been absorbed by the scalp.

This is a mechanical problem, not a blood supply problem. The skills required to manage this problem well take years to learn; it is for this reason that dense packing is not widely accepted.

Figure 16–3. See the healed grafts in the scalp and the new grafts added in a second session, thereby doubling density.

Through a series of such procedures, successive groups of small grafts (1-4 hairs) are placed in a way that creates a dense appearing hairline with a normal, soft transition that frames the face. To appear natural, grafts must be graded with 1-hair units in the leading edge and larger units behind the leading edge.

# 17

## THE PSYCHOLOGY OF HAIR RESTORATION PATIENTS

Men under the age of 25 with hair loss are having hair restoration procedures more frequently today. These young men are confronted by both their entry into manhood and the perception that their balding is aging them at an accelerated rate. These patients often feel deprived of an essential element of their youth. This feeling is created and affirmed, seemingly by everything our western culture promotes.

Hair is indicative of a healthy, youthful appearance. Images on television and in the movies reinforce the association between a youthful appearance and a full head of hair. It is difficult for a young man who is balding to sort out his identity when surrounded by a world of hairy, virile, healthy, "normal" appearing young men. For these young hair transplant candidates, objectivity does not always prevail. Panic sometimes generates the decision to get their hair back. The premature loss of hair becomes equated, in their minds, with the premature loss of their youth; therefore, medical education, ethics, and honest rules of engagement (informed consent) must be high on the physician's priorities when discussing the hair restoration procedure with this youthful subset of the balding population.

Men in their 30's and early 40's are more deliberate about the decision to undergo hair transplant surgery. Many have considered the procedure for some time, but faced with the difficulty of getting accurate information and finding a doctor they trust, they may wisely delay the decision. Some outside factor may finally push them to become serious in pursuing hair restoration surgery. This factor may be a business decision, (a younger looking person may have more earning potential), a divorce, or the availability of financial resources.

Alternatively, it may reflect the self-indulgence of a confident, successful person doing something for himself.

Having hair restoration surgery is moderately expensive. The cost depends upon several factors: the amount of work that must be done based upon the level of hair loss, the expectations of the patient, the proposed method, and who will perform the work. It may cost more than a mid-size car, a cruise, or a safari, so it deserves serious consideration. A vacation or a safari lasts but a few weeks; a mid-sized car will last a few years; but a hair restoration will last a lot longer. The cost of the restoration is a factor, but should not be the overwhelming determinant.

Going to an expensive surgeon does not guarantee good results. If the cost of the work exceeds the patient's ability to pay for what he actually needs, the patient may not be able to finish the work he started. A poorly planned procedure, or failure to complete what was started, can produce a medical oddity. A properly staged procedure over long periods is as good a choice as a Fast Track® approach. The key to a successful hair restoration is the creation of a customized plan that reflects the goals of each patient. An attempt to cut costs can lead to a lifetime of regret every time you look in the mirror. One should ask: "How much hair will I actually get for the dollars I am planning to spend?" As men grow older, they become more discriminating. They have life experience, and know what they want because they have the maturity to make balanced, non-emotional judgments. They are thoughtful about the decision process and they usually take the time to research their choices reasonably well. For those who can afford it, there is no substitute for the best money can buy. Men under 30 may be more motivated by the emotional aspect of looking older too soon. They are vulnerable to high-pressure sales tactics by unscrupulous salesmen. Men over 30 often feel they have worked hard, achieved a great deal and therefore decide to reward themselves. More often, they may want to look as young as they feel, and having hair is important to their sense of well being.

# 18

## DETERMINING QUALITY AND VALUE

### Quality

Quality in hair transplantation is priceless and although we often tie quality, value, and price together; quality should never be compromised. Small, delicate grafts are critical to high quality results in hair transplantation. Value must be judged by evaluating both quality and cost. When comparing the cost of procedures offered by different medical groups, it must be an apples-to-apples comparison. Ask:

- How many grafts will I receive in each session? What is the size of the grafts and how many hairs will each graft contain? How many hairs will be moved in each session?

- Will I have sufficient donor hair after completion of this procedure for future hair restoration?

- How much will I pay for each graft in each session? How many sessions will I need? What can I expect to pay for the entire hair restoration process?

Your goal should be to achieve the best quality work with the highest number of hairs moved in the smallest, most practical graft size. One hair at a time may produce inadequate density. Naturally appearing follicular unit grafts of 1-4 hairs may make more sense. When hairs are clumped together in unnatural groupings, there may be a lower initial cost, but these hair transplants will be detectable to the naked eye (toothbrush look) and an unnecessarily rapid depletion of your remaining donor hair as more hair is moved in this way. It is critically important to recognize that compromise may be necessary, and each patient must be in a position to understand the benefits and liabilities of each element in the decision process when planning the size and distribution of the transplants.

The larger the size of your grafts, the more hairs will be in each graft and the more unnatural you will look as these larger grafts produce a greater contrast to the surrounding skin. Larger grafts also tend to be more wasteful and deplete the donor supply faster than smaller grafts. Smaller grafts appear more natural, but they may have a smaller impact on the balding area if they are not done in substantial quantities.

## Negative Value

Having an unnatural appearance, spending money out of proportion to the benefits you receive, losing valuable time in living a normal life, and accelerating the hair loss process, are all signs of negative value. Deciding whether to have hair restoration and what type of hair restoration to have is difficult, and your time investment must be part of the formula and multiple small surgeries take a high toll on the patient in many ways.

The worst outcome possible occurs in the patient who receives poor quality work that cannot be fully corrected. The negative value is incalculable, as the patient may have to live with the consequences of this error for the rest of his or her life. For a person who undertook the hair restoration process to avoid a wig, wearing one to cover a bad job is a daily reminder of his or her mistake. A toothbrush appearance often takes more work and more money to fix than it took to create, if surgical corrections are possible at all. In these situations, the cost may sharply increase in trying to correct what cannot truly be repaired. Camouflage is the only answer and is always imperfect.

## Value

How do you determine value of a purchase of this magnitude and of such a personal nature? This issue needs to be answered to the comfort of each individual patient before making the decision to have any hair restoration or transplant procedure. Value is determined by such factors as:

1. Your results will reflect the outcome after your work is complete and all of your transplanted hair has grown in. A true understanding of the value of your surgery cannot be assessed until after the work is complete. You should compare what was anticipated with what was achieved and the two should approximate each other. As having hair will give you a different perspective, it is important to make this comparison relative to your starting point, as your memory may fade and your mind may repress any connection with your old bald or thin look.

2. Inconvenience reflects the time you dedicated to the hair restoration process at the expense of work, the discomfort associated with each procedure, the social dislocations caused by each procedure, etc. If you feel that your hair restoration has been of value, that value will tend to minimize these inconveniences. To properly estimate the inconveniences involved in surgical hair restoration, you should personally interview some of your proposed doctor's patients. Their experiences will act as a reality check on what the doctor told you. This should be done before the surgical process is started.

3. Risk reflects all of the uncertainties (real or imagined) including medical complications of the procedures, psychological ramifications associated with the process, and social effects before, during, and after transplantation. Proper research and interviews with patients will address these issues in advance.

4. The total cost of the process in terms of lost time at work, opportunity costs, social costs, and total dollars spent must be related to the results you achieved. Such measurements as cost per session, cost per graft, cost per

transferred hair follicle and the like, reflect value in measurable units. The ability of your surgeon to accurately estimate the cost of a restoration should be anticipated before a procedure is begun. Meet with patients who have had extensive reconstructions by the doctor you are going to choose. Lowballing is more common than anyone is willing to admit. Do not get suckered into a false sense of security without proper interviews with some of the doctor's previous patients.

5.  Commitment to completion means that the question that must be asked is: "must I complete the process once start ed?" Well-performed minigrafts or Follicular Unit Grafts, when done correctly in accordance to a customized Master Plan (depending upon hair character and color), will allow each session to stand independent of every other session, achieving in the worst case a thinner appearance than was originally planned. Ask the doctor if one procedure can stand on its own.

6.  Time from start to end of procedures reflects not only the calendar months from the first to the last procedure, but also the number of surgeries required to reach the last procedure. Each surgery produces down time, social dislocations, possibly lost time at work, some level of physical discomfort and considerable anxiety. The time span for all this may be months or years in some Master Plans.

These six areas are critical in order to understand value. In the final measurement, only results count. A pluggy appearance will have a negative value for most people. A thin natural look may only have partial value if the patient was expecting a full head of hair. On the other hand, a thin look may be the only reasonable expectation for a person with advanced baldness, high contrast of skin to hair color, straight fine hair or a limited supply of hair. Evaluation of your results must relate your gains after surgery to the expectations established at the onset of the process.

# 19

## HAIR LOSS IN WOMEN

Until now, this discussion has been confined primarily to the effects and treatment of hair loss in men. Men were the first patients to have hair transplants, and men comprise about 98% of hair all transplantation patients today. Several factors may play a part in this phenomenon. In the past, baldness was usually portrayed as an exclusively male phenomenon. After the 1700's, men stopped wearing wigs over full heads of hair, but women have continued to wear wigs and hairpieces. Women wear wigs not only to compensate for hair loss, but also to change their hairstyles or color, to conceal bad haircuts and make dramatic fashion statements. Advertising and research about hair replacement has almost exclusively addressed the problem in men. It is important, however, to be aware that, though men are usually the ones recognized as having hair loss, and though the hair loss process is commonly called male pattern baldness, women are also affected by androgenetic alopecia. Women represent 40% of the U.S. balding or thinning population, but their hair loss tends to manifest itself in overall thinning of the hair, including thinning of the donor area. It is the stable donor area that, in male patients, makes successful hair transplantation possible. Unfortunately, seventy-five percent of women with androgenetic alopecia may not be suitable candidates for hair transplantation.

Many women come to a hair transplant surgeon as a last resort. Most are desperate, as the medical community ignores their complaints about hair loss. Successful female hair transplant candidates must be healthy, have no evidence of thyroid disease and their hormonal history must be taken. Prior to hair transplantation surgery, the following conditions should be considered as possible causes of female hair loss: anemia, thyroid disease, connective tissue disease, gynecological conditions and emotional stress. It is also important to review the use of medications that can cause hair loss, such as oral contraceptives, beta-blockers, vitamin A, thyroid drugs, coumadin and prednisone. The following laboratory tests are often useful if underlying problems are suspected: CBC, Chem Screen, ANA, T4, TSH, STS, Androstenedione, DHEA-Sulfate, Total and Free Testosterone. Once these medical conditions are eliminated as possible causes of female hair loss, genetics is the most common cause of the balding or thinning process. Women who are candidates for hair transplantation usually have widespread, generalized thinning; and they want widespread generalized thickening, so an education in realistic expectations is critical.

Female androgenetic alopecia is generally observed as an intact frontal 1/3rd inch of hairline while the area behind this "permanent" hairline is thinning or balding. A full and careful examination of the scalp is essential in making the correct diagnosis. The proper diagnosis of the female patient with hair loss is a critical step in assessing which women can be helped by hair transplantation and which women may be further damaged by the hair transplantation process. Chemically, testosterone is related to the two major female sex hormones: estrogen and progesterone. A portion of the estrogen circulating in a woman's body is normally converted into a hormone that has male sex hormone activity. This process is more active in elderly and obese women. This helps to explain why some older and overweight women have more facial and body hair than others.

Men tend to wear shorter hairstyles than most women do. Transplanted hair, like natural hair, grows at a rate of about 1 cm (0.5 inches) per month. For most men, transplanted hair reaches a length where it adds additional bulk to the background hair within 3-6 months. For women, this same process often takes 12 months because of the greater length of the background hair. Female patients have a difficult time seeing the growth during this interim. No matter how often they are reassured, many female patients may become discouraged.

Despite these problems, women make excellent hair replacement patients. Many of the problems that men experience do not occur in women. Women's hair is often longer than men's hair; therefore, immediate coverage of the donor area is not usually a problem. While visualization of the additional bulk of new hair takes more time in women than it does in men, women do not have the problem of visibility of the grafts that bald men do. Women who are losing their hair tend to style the remaining hair long enough to provide some coverage of the balding area. This coverage also hides the new grafts while they are growing in. This allows denser placement of grafts in the initial procedure, and may reduce the total number of hair transplant sessions. This same factor also allows a woman to schedule treatment sessions at longer intervals than is usual for men.

Many women who have had face lift surgery are left with a band of scar that runs from just in front of one ear across the top of the head to the opposite side. The central part of this scar is easily concealed by long hair, but the scar just in front of the ears is harder to hide. Women who have this problem must adapt their hairstyles to cover the scars. Unfortunately, most women and many doctors are not aware that the central part of the scar can be reduced in a simple office procedure and the scar in front of the ears can be completely replaced with hair transplants that have a natural appearance.

Traction alopecia is a form of hair loss almost unique to women. Traction alopecia can result in recession of the hairline when hair is chronically pulled very tight to form braids or pigtails. In the United States, it is most commonly seen in

African American women. This type of hair loss can often be corrected with transplants.

## The Key is Diagnosis

The degree of miniaturization of hair follicles must be assessed throughout the scalp. This assessment is critical in qualifying women for surgery. In males, miniaturization is usually localized in the balding pattern. In women, the miniaturization of hair may be localized (as in males) or it may extend over the entire scalp, including part or all of the fringe area around the sides and the back of the head. The first step in deciding whether a woman is a candidate for transplantation should be to assess the degree of miniaturization throughout the scalp. Women whose entire "fringe" areas show significant miniaturization are generally not good candidates for hair transplantation. For women with limited "permanent" zone involvement, it may be possible to perform a transplant providing that their expectations are realistic. Telogen effluvium (short term hair loss caused by surgical trauma to hair follicles) is common after hair transplantation procedures in women.

Hair transplantation should be viewed as a localized process for most female patients. Transplantation can be quite beneficial when used to augment styling in the front, where the hair is parted, or in a local, well-defined area where styling is difficult such as a side or midline part. Treatment of women who qualify for hair transplantation falls into four categories:

- A woman with a loss pattern similar to a man can be treated in a manner similar to the approach we use with men if the "permanent" zone does not show significant miniaturization.
- A woman who maintains her original frontal hairline with balding or thinning behind it, can often be treated by adding density to create fullness in defined areas.

- A woman who has generalized thinning in the front, top and crown areas can have added density if the entire "permanent" zone is not impacted by the miniaturization process. The density should be designed to augment styling, not solve the thinning problem.
- A woman who has lost hair secondary to another cosmetic procedure such as a facelift or brow-lift may be a good candidate for hair transplant surgery. The complications of facial surgery are compounded by scars either at the hairline or behind it. Side hairlines (including sideburns) can be satisfactorily transplanted.

The art and science of women's hair restoration is distinctly different from men's. Widespread ignorance is pervasive in the medical profession, and few medical articles address hair transplantation for women. It is critical that the doctor first rule out underlining systemic disease (thyroid disease, collagen vascular disease, anemia, etc.) and the various causes of telogen effluvium (weight loss, pregnancy, oral contraceptives and stress), which are reversible over time. A thorough family history usually demonstrates similar genetic patterns in mothers or siblings. Women who are candidates for hair transplantation are among the most satisfied patients we treat.

# 20

## REPAIRING BAD HAIR TRANSPLANTS

A significant number of hair restoration surgeries performed at the New Hair Institute involve some type of corrective procedures to fix bad hair transplants, scalp reductions and flaps performed by other physicians. The following describes the approach that NHI physicians use when dealing with patients who need repair work.

Improperly performed hair restoration surgeries present a series of unique problems that often must be solved by deviating from the normal rules that would apply to performing a hair transplant on a "virgin" scalp. Repairs require far more experience and creativity on the part of the surgeon than when performing the original transplant. In repair procedures, the surgeon encounters a multitude of problems that often exist simultaneously. Unfortunately, the improper techniques that cause the cosmetic defects are often the same ones that limit the repair. Fundamental to all repair work, therefore, is establishing a series of goals that are carefully prioritized so that, in the event they cannot all be met, the ones most critical to the patient's appearance are dealt with first.

The patient who has had a bad hair transplant experience is often depressed, angry and distrusting. Therefore, the surgeon attempting a repair has a number of challenges, not all surgical. He must restore confidence in a patient who feels he was betrayed by the medical establishment and who often wishes he had never started with the hair restoration process in the first place. The physician must establish trust in a patient who had been misled, establish new goals when previous goals had not been met, and explain a sequence of new procedures when the prior ones were not well understood. The doctor must also convince his patient to embark on a new series of surgeries with the understanding that obvious benefit may not be apparent after the initial procedures. He must plan his surgery in concert with the social needs of the patient and design the procedure so that specific styling and grooming techniques can be used to enhance the surgery. The doctor must then perform surgery with techniques individualized to the particular patient and deal with problems that cannot always be anticipated before the surgery is begun. Restoration work is a creative endeavor that combines communication, surgical and aesthetic skills to achieve the patient's goals.

Although many problem results reflect procedures that were routinely performed prior to the advent of the use of small grafts, the availability of "modern techniques" alone does not protect the patient against bad work. Errors in surgical and aesthetic judgment, performing procedures on non-candidates, and operating on patients with unrealistic expectations, still remain major problems. Therefore, extreme care in selecting a surgeon is just as important today even though, as a whole, physicians are performing better surgery.

The use of very small grafts, and now follicular unit grafts, eliminates many of the more blatant problems associated with the older procedures. However, there are "cost cutting" techniques used by some physicians that create new areas of concern. One of these is the automated "graft cutter" where thin slivers of donor tissue are placed on a series of blades and smacked with a hammer into smaller pieces. These techniques appear to save the patient money, however, they unnecessarily destroy precious donor hair and limit the amount of fullness that can be achieved. Even procedures touted as state-of-the-art technology, such as laser hair transplantation, can cause harm to unwary patients by slowing the healing process and causing unnecessary scarring in the recipient area.

## Problems Seen with Bad Hair Transplants

The major cosmetic problems encountered with poorly planned, or improperly executed, hair restoration surgery can be classified as follows:

- Grafts too large or "pluggy";
- Hairline too far forward;
- Hairline too broad;
- Hair placed in the wrong direction;
- Unrealistic area of attempted coverage;
- Scarring in the recipient area;
- Ridging;
- Hair wastage; and
- Donor area scarring.

Many of these problems are interrelated and patients needing repair work often have multiple problems to correct. Before "correcting" an old transplant, it is important to first establish what aspects of the old work bother the patient most. The patient must clearly express his or her concerns and his or her priorities, and then discuss the management of each of these issues with the physician. It may not always be possible to solve all the problems, but partial improvement may still be a worthy goal. Some aspects of the transplant that bother the surgeon may be left untreated if they do not necessarily concern the patient. Setting priorities before the repair has begun will help ensure maximum patient satisfaction.

## Large Grafts

There are multiple problems with patients who have received larger grafts. When hair is distributed properly in a hair restoration procedure, the density should not exceed 50% of one's original density. The reason for this is that the normal human scalp has at least a 100% visual redundancy. This means that the eye cannot perceive hair loss until it exceeds 50%. There is, then, no logical reason to restore more than

50%, especially in view of the fact that the balding individual has less total hair volume.

As a result of the contraction of plugs once they have been transplanted, the density of hair in the plugs may actually exceed the donor density. This produces a pattern of excessive density within the larger grafts and empty spaces between them. In most patients who will have a significant amount of balding, there is not enough donor hair to both fill in the spaces between the plugs and cover all the area that needs to have hair. As a result, the surgeon is left with the dilemma of choosing between a pluggy look scattered over a large area or very high density in some areas with insufficient coverage in others. Often the patient is left with both problems!

It is important to note that one often observes less density in the grafts than one would anticipate from the size of the harvested plug. This can be due to a number of different mechanisms. Two of the most common are hair loss from poor harvesting techniques, and hair loss caused by a phenomenon called "doughnutting." In doughnutting, the centers of grafts get insufficient oxygen following transplantation and therefore, the follicles in the central portion of the grafts fail to survive. This results in hair growing only in the periphery of the grafts. This was a common phenomenon in 4- and 5-mm plugs, but can also be noted in grafts 3-mm in size. A "crescent moon" deformity occurs when these two problems exist simultaneously and the transection, in effect, cuts off half of the doughnut leaving a crescent moon shape. An additional problem is that, in these cases, even though the appearance might not be very pluggy, the total available donor hair is markedly decreased. These problems do not occur with micrografts or follicular unit grafts.

## A Hairline that is Too Low or Too Broad

Although the adolescent hairline hugs the upper brow crease, the position of the normal adult male hairline is approximately one fingerbreadth higher (1.5 cm above the upper brow crease at the midline). A common mistake of the inexperienced hair restoration surgeon is to restore the hairline to the adolescent, rather than the normal adult position. Hairlines that have been restored to the low adolescent position are most commonly seen in younger patients whose memory of their adolescent hairline is still fresh in their minds and who put considerable pressure on the doctor to place hair in this location. Unfortunately, this also occurs in the situation where the physician is anxious to get the patient "started" with surgery rather than embarking on a more conservative (and more appropriate) medical treatment. A low frontal hairline not only distorts the patient's facial proportions, it sets expectations that are unsustainable if the balding progresses, and precludes a natural balanced look to the restoration as the patient ages.

## Hair Placed in the Wrong Direction

In the front and top part of the scalp hair grows in a distinctly forward direction changing to a circular pattern, only as one approaches the crown. The hair always emerges from the scalp at an acute angle, with the angle being most acute at the temples. The patient's own hair direction must be followed exactly if there is any hope of the transplant looking natural. The only exception would be with swirls at the frontal hairline that most likely won't be permanent.

Unfortunately, there has been a tendency for hair restoration surgeons, using larger grafts, to transplant them perpendicular to the skin from the outset. This is probably due to the fact that the mechanics of the old plug procedures made sharp angling technically difficult and resulted in more elevation and/or pitting when the grafts healed. Sadly, these habits persist even with the use of very small grafts. It is not uncommon to see a patient whose transplanted frontal hairline has hair pointing in a radial direction, giving a "Statue of Liberty" appearance. Another problem with placing hair perpendicular to the scalp is that the viewer looks into the base of the hair shaft (where the hair inserts into the scalp). This looks distinctly abnormal, although the patient is often unaware of the problem. In a properly performed hair transplant, the hair is transplanted pointing forward and then when the hair is groomed to the side or back, the hair is bent (bowed), showing the curve of the hair shaft to the viewer, rather than the base.

## Unrealistic Area of Attempted Coverage

The first area to bald is generally the area where you should be most wary when transplanting. This useful guideline is commonly ignored by doctors anxious to get their patients started with surgery. For example, the temples and crown generally bald first, but recession at the temples and thinning in the crown are very acceptable, especially as the patient ages. The central forelock region, however, is generally late to bald (particularly in certain family lines), but when it is lost, the patient looses the frame to his face and its restoration becomes essential.

An adequate amount of hair must always be reserved for the critical areas such as the forelock and top of the scalp, regardless of whether these areas need coverage at the time of the initial transplant. If the patient's donor reserves are limited, due to poor scalp laxity, low donor density, fine hair shaft diameter or a host of other reasons, the transplantation of other less critical areas should be postponed or avoided entirely. A pattern that resembles "two horns and a tail" may result when doctors are too aggressive in transplanting the temples and crown in a young person. This can become a cosmetic nightmare for the patent when there is further balding and these regions cannot be connected due to inadequate donor reserves.

## Scarring in the Recipient Area

Traditional round grafts require the largest wounds, but even mini-micrografting produces wounds that can be unnecessarily large as most of the donor tissue is transplanted along with the hair. These large wounds often result in scarring. Scarring has a number of undesirable effects on the transplant. When severe, it can cause graft elevation or depression, loss of grafts after the surgery and poor hair growth. When mild, scarring may result in subtle textural and visual irregularities in the skin around the grafts, produce a distortion of the hair direction and cause a change in quality of the hair shaft, all reducing the chance of a cosmetically satisfactory result.

Laser hair transplantation, more aptly termed "laser site creation" represents the epitome of purposeless scarring. The laser itself is nothing more than a marketing gimmick. Basically, the laser is a glorified "punch" that creates holes or slits in the recipient scalp by removing (vaporizing) tissue. The laser is smartly marketed with claims that "the beam is so precise that the zone of thermal injury can be measured in microns." However, regardless of how little damage is done to surrounding tissue, the recipient tissue directly under the beam is totally destroyed.

The laser has the additional disadvantages of increased set-up time, greater cost, and potential eye hazards. The laser operator lacks the precise tactile and visual guidance to adjust for depth and angle when making sites on a curved scalp. Most important, the laser destroys tissue and unnecessarily increases the recipient wound size.

## Ridging

Another significant cosmetic problem produced by larger grafts is the extra volume of tissue introduced into the recipient site. This extra tissue produces a fullness and elevation of the transplanted area and a clinically apparent ridge, separating it from the surrounding bald scalp. In some patients, this problem is compounded by a negative reaction of the surrounding tissue in response to the transplanted grafts. This phenomenon, termed "hyperfibrotic change" by Dr. Dow Stough, accentuates the abnormal contour of the transplanted area. In addition, there is some evidence that the hair subsequently placed into this area may exhibit sub-optimal growth.

Hyperfibrotic changes are rarely seen with very small grafts and have not been reported with Follicular Unit Transplantation.

## Wasting Hair

Wastage of donor hair, not often noted initially, is a major limitation to preserving adequate density for sufficient coverage. It is the hidden enemy of all successful repairs. Hair wastage comes in many forms: poor graft harvesting and dissection, improper graft storage and handling, keeping the grafts out of the body too long, packing the transplanted grafts too closely in the scalp, poor pre-operative preparation, or inadequate post-op care. Literally every step of a poorly executed transplant may serve to deplete one's donor supply.

An interesting paradox occurs with the old punch-graft technique. When the procedure is executed flawlessly, most of the donor hair is captured in each punch and the growth of the grafts appears pluggy, inciting immediate complaints on the part of the patient. When the procedure is performed poorly, there is increased transection of the harvested follicles and inadequate growth in the centers of the larger grafts, both contributing to a softer, more natural look. Although in the latter situation, the patients are initially more satisfied, the poor growth is evidence that there will be problems with hair supply down the line and, ultimately, a worse cosmetic result.

## Donor Scarring

Although the major effect of scarring in the donor area is to decrease the amount of available hair, when scarring is severe, the scar itself may become a cosmetic problem. The situations where this is most likely to occur are when the scar is: placed too high (in the non-permanent zone), placed too low (near the nape of the neck or over the ear), excessively wide in any location, or raised (a hypertrophic scar or a keloid).

## Limiting Factor in Repair Procedures

Many of the cosmetic defects created by poor techniques can be completely reversed or "partially undone" by meticulously removing and re-implanting unsightly grafts. However, the main factor that often prevents the surgeon from achieving all of the patient's restorative goals is a limited donor supply.

Hair wastage due to poor surgical techniques is usually the main cause of this donor supply depletion. The early telltale signs of hair wastage may be a transplant that appears too thin for the number of grafts used, poor growth manifested as gaps at the hairline, or uneven density in areas where the coverage should be uniform. The fact that donor hair was wasted might be surmised from a longer donor incision than one would expect for a given number of grafts, or abnormally low density in the donor area in the vicinity of the donor scar. Unfortunately, it is very difficult to ascertain exactly what the underlying causes had been after the fact and, by the time surgeon is aware that he has run out of usable donor hair, the damage has already been done.

Because adequate donor supply is so critical to a successful repair, accurately assessing the amount of hair available becomes paramount. When performing a hair transplant on a virgin scalp, quantifying the donor supply is rather straightforward, since the density and scalp laxity are relatively uniform in the donor area. In repairs, however, additional factors come into play, so that even though there might appear to be enough hair in the donor area, it might not be available to the surgeon for use. Factors that limit the available donor hair include:

- Low donor density,
- Fine hair caliber,
- Poor scalp mobility, and
- Scarring.

## Low Donor Density

Donor hair density can be measured using a simple handheld device called a Densitometer. The average Caucasian has approximately 2.0 hairs/mm$^2$, but this can vary from as little as 1.5 hairs/mm$^2$ to greater than 3 hairs/mm$^2$. In most individuals, the density of follicular units in one's scalp (follicular unit density) is relatively constant at 1 follicular unit/mm$^2$. After hair transplantation procedures, the average density in the donor area decreases. Unfortunately, after poor hair transplant surgery, there isn't a corresponding increase in hair in the recipient areas of the scalp.

In modern strip harvesting, the resulting linear scar gives little indication of the strip's actual size, as it only reflects the length of the excised strip and not its width. Thus, the actual amount of tissue that had been removed cannot readily be ascertained.

Using densitometry, this information can be measured by looking at the increased spacing of follicular units. The percent of measured decrease in follicular unit density will give an indication of how much tissue had been removed and more important, how much is left to harvest. You cannot obtain this information from measuring hair density alone if it had not been measured before the surgery. Unfortunately, doctors who perform bad hair transplants rarely pay attention to measuring hair density, and even less commonly record it in the patient's file.

## Fine Hair Caliber

Although not affected by the transplant, hair shaft diameter is an extremely important contributor to hair volume and thus the available hair supply. Hair shaft diameter is mentioned less often than the actual number of hairs because it is more difficult to measure, but its importance to both the virgin transplant and to a repair cannot be overemphasized. Variations in hair shaft diameter have an approximately 2.7 times greater impact on the appearance of fullness than the absolute number of hairs.

The importance of this in a repair is that, for a given degree of plugginess, fine hair will provide less camouflage than coarser hair. Fine hair, therefore, must be transplanted in greater numbers, or in multiple sessions, to achieve the same results. When this quantity of hair is not available, compromises must be made in the repair. This important issue should be discussed with patients who have fine hair prior to the repair, so that priorities can be established in advance.

## Poor Scalp Mobility

Donor density and hair shaft diameter are not the only factors affecting the available donor supply. In order for an adequate amount of hair to be harvested, there needs to be sufficient scalp laxity (looseness) to close the wound after the donor strip is removed. Especially when there is low donor density, having adequate laxity is especially important because a widened scar may be visible through the thin hair. The location of the donor incision greatly affects scalp mobility. The ideal position for the donor incision is in the mid-portion of the permanent zone. The muscles of the neck insert into the deeper tissues of the scalp just below that area. The problem is that an incision placed below this area will be affected by the muscle movement directly beneath it. A stretched scar in this location is extremely difficult to repair since re-excision, even with undermining and layered closure, will tend to heal with an even wider scar.

The main risk of placing the scars too high is the lack of permanence of the transplanted hair (it may be subject to androgenetic alopecia), and future visibility of the scar if the donor fringe were to narrow further.

## Scarring

Scarring in the donor area limits the amount of hair accessible to the surgeon for a number of reasons. The most obvious reason is that a larger donor strip must be removed to harvest the same amount of hair. The second, mentioned above, is that scarring decreases scalp laxity by destroying elastic tissue and often destroying the subcutaneous layer causing the scalp skin to be bound down to the deeper tissues. The third is that scars themselves present cosmetic problems when visible, so more donor hair must be left to cover a scarred area than to cover normal scalp.

The presence of open donor scars, made by the old punch technique may give a false sense of security. Because an excision with a primary closure was not performed, the patient's donor laxity has not been compromised. This thinking may lure the unwary surgeon into harvesting a donor strip that is too wide. When the surgeon attempts to close the donor wound, the tight closure requires more tension on the sutures. The sutures, however, tend to tear the scarred wound edges (that are significantly more fragile and inflexible than normal scalp), increasing the scarring and hindering the repair.

## Follicular Unit Transplantation: The Ideal Tool for Repair

Poor planning, bad judgment and sloppy techniques in hair transplantation result in cosmetic defects and poor hair growth. Some of the problems with a hair transplant, however, are intrinsic to the procedure and cannot be completely avoided, regardless of how conscientious the doctor or impeccable the technique. This is because even moderately sized grafts run the risk of scarring and an uneven appearance.

To avoid these problems, NHI Physicians advise performing the entire hair restoration procedure using exclusively follicular units. In repair procedures where there is already scarring and hair wastage, using a procedure that minimizes wounds, maximizes the utilization of donor hair, and looks totally natural, is even more important. Follicular Unit Transplantation is the ideal tool for the following four reasons:

- The techniques used in FUT, namely single strip harvesting and microscopic dissection, insure maximum utilization of the donor supply.
- The small size of follicular units permits small wounds that limit further damage to areas that have already been scarred.
- The relatively greater hair content of follicular units, as compared to mini-micrografts of the same size, allows them to provide greater camouflage.
- Follicular unit grafts duplicate the way hair grows in nature and therefore provide the most natural restoration.

Excising the donor tissue as a single strip is especially important in repair work since the orientation of hair follicles in the donor scalp has been altered from prior surgery. Because of this, a multi-bladed knife (the traditional harvesting tool in mini-micrografting) can cause excessive follicular transection. Once the strip is removed, microscopic dissection allows for the retrieval of donor hair in, and around, the scar tissue produced by the old transplants, significantly increasing the amount of usable hair. Traditional graft dissection, without the use of a microscope, does not provide enough resolution to ensure that the follicles, distorted by the surrounding scar tissue, are removed intact.

When follicular units are dissected from the donor strip, grafts are generated that contain a greater proportion of hair in relation to skin than in the surrounding tissue. This is unique in hair restoration surgery as both punch grafts and mini-micrografts have essentially the same ratio of skin and hair as the tissue from which they were derived. Since the follicular unit is a more compact hair-bearing structure, it can fit into smaller recipient wounds (minimizing additional insult to the donor area) and provide for greater coverage (or camouflage of poor work). In addition, since follicular unit grafts mimic the way hair grows in nature, it is logical to take advantage of them in hair restoration.

## Repair Strategies

There are two basic repair strategies that are often used in conjunction with one another: removal with re-implantation of the grafts and camouflage. In the following sections, specific techniques will be grouped under these broad strategies.

Camouflage is the primary means used to improve the cosmetic appearance of a poorly executed transplant. In this situation, the existing grafts are used to provide volume or bulk to the transplant. The camouflage, small mini-micrografts or follicular units, is used to create a more natural appearance. When possible, camouflage should be used as the sole restorative procedure since excision and re-implantation require extra procedures and will postpone the completion of the restoration. In addition, the process of removing grafts may cause some damage to the hair follicles and produce additional scarring. Since removal of large numbers of grafts may result in less total hair volume, they should not be removed indiscriminately.

Camouflage should be preceded by excision and re-implantation when camouflage alone is incapable of producing a satisfactory result. This usually occurs when:

1. The existing grafts are too large to be camouflaged.
2. There are grafts in an inappropriate location.
    • The hairline is too low or too broad.

- The temples have been inappropriately transplanted.
- The crown has been transplanted in the face of an inadequate donor supply.

3.  The hair direction is wrong.

When grafts are too large, in a position where placing additional grafts in front of them would bring the hairline down too low, when the hair that they contain is pointing in the wrong direction, or when the grafts are simply in an area that should not have been transplanted, their removal is mandatory. Camouflage alone in these situations will likely exaggerate an already unacceptable appearance.

If excision and re-implantation are indicated, they should be performed before the camouflage is undertaken to achieve the best possible results. Once additional grafts have been placed, removing the old ones becomes much more problematic and additional hair wastage and scarring result. When in doubt, it is best to err on the side of removing inappropriately placed grafts, rather that trying to cover them up.

The traditional approach to improving the appearance of plugs is to attempt to fill in the empty spaces between the grafts with additional large grafts. The main problem with this method is that it takes an area of already high density and makes it even greater. Since the resultant density is impossible to sustain, the patient runs a serious risk of completely depleting his donor reserves. This, in turn, forces the surgeon into leaving gaps in the area being fixed, and leaving other cosmetically important areas uncovered. Another problem is that the use of large grafts in the repair produces additional scarring (and decreased blood supply in an area already markedly scarred). As a result, not only may the new grafts exhibit poor growth, but they decrease the chance that future procedures will be successful.

A preferred approach to improving the appearance of plugs is to reduce the density of these larger grafts by excising a portion of them and then redistributing the hair obtained from immediate.

When the main cosmetic problem is that the plugs are too large or dense, the goal may be to simply decrease their density rather than to remove them completely. In this situation, the splay of follicles below the surface of the skin will permit some hair to remain in the area even if all of the hair visible on the surface appears to have been removed. As a general guide, we find that approximately 25% of the hair in most punches will re-grow even if the punch fits neatly over all of the emerging hair.

With grafts behind the hairline, one should only remove enough hair so that they can be camouflaged in subsequent sessions. The decision regarding how much of the grafts should actually be removed will depend upon both the grafts themselves and also the patient's donor reserves. With high donor reserves and centrally placed grafts, little density reduction is usually required, even if the grafts are large. However, in patients with depleted donor reserves where significant camouflage is not possible, the visual impact of these grafts often needs to be completely neutralized with excision and re-implantation.

Grafts at or near the frontal hairline almost always need to be reduced to 1-3 hairs to look natural after a camouflage. In spite of the relative ease of removing only part of a graft, all of the hair in the graft should be completely removed if: 1) the grafts are in an inappropriate location, i.e. too low on the forehead or in the temples or crown, 2) when it is not appropriate to transplant in affected areas, or 3) the hair has been transplanted pointing in the wrong direction. When the grafts are to be removed entirely, it is extremely important to tell the patient that this will most likely require more than one session, as some re-growth of hair is the rule, rather than the exception.

Excised grafts are immediately placed under a stereomicroscope and dissected into individual follicular units. In the these grafts into an adjacent area (as individual follicular units). This will decrease the density of the problem area and permit additional areas to be transplanted with less density, since the potential contrast will have been reduced. This, in turn will produce a more balanced look and conserve donor hair.

## Repair Techniques

Graft removal with re-implantation of the hair as individual follicular units, and camouflage can be used for most restorative work. As discussed above, these can be used alone or in conjunction with one another.

- Removal and Re-implantation
- Punch excision
- Linear excision
- Electrolysis
- Laser Hair Removal
- Camouflage
- Concept of Camouflage
- Establishing the Frontal Hairline
- Transition Zones
- Angling
- Forward and Side Weighting
- The Hockey Stick
- Carpet Tacking

## Punch Excision

Removing part of a large graft is a simple technique that can be used to decrease the unnatural density of the old plugs. It is accomplished by punching or "coring out," part of the old graft and leaving a crescent shaped section of hair behind. This method has a number of advantages: 1) it preserves some of the hair in the original graft, 2) it enables the removed hair to be re-used, 3) it can remove and improve the appearance of some of the scarred underlying skin and, 4) its results are average repair case performed in our office, one excised graft yields approximately 3-4 follicular units, although usually not all of the units are intact because of the damage caused by the original procedure(s). The new follicular unit grafts are placed in a region of hair loss separate from the area of plug removal.

It is important not to plant the new grafts too closely together, since repair surgeries are best spaced only two months apart, giving insufficient time for the hair to grow to a visible length before the next procedure. By spreading out the small number of follicular grafts harvested from plugs over a relatively large area, it is unlikely that grafts of a subsequent session will interfere with those of the first, even if placed in the same location.

It is usually difficult to remove multiple rows of closely spaced grafts in one session as the closure of one wound may place tension on the next, especially if the grafts are in adjacent rows. This is less of a problem when removing adjacent grafts in a linear arrangement, since, in this situation, the closure of one graft has little impact on an adjacent one, and may even make the subsequent closure easier. When the removal of one graft interferes with the next, then every other graft should be removed and the restoration should be carried out in multiple sessions.

The majority of patients require 1-3 sessions of graft removal prior to the actual camouflage procedure. There should be a two-month interval between graft excisions and a two-month interval between the last excision and the actual camouflage. The period between repairs allows hair in the grafts to grow so that the visible stubble may direct the removal of residual hair in previously excised grafts. The two-month period between the last excision and the camouflage allows the sutured area to heal well enough that it will accept new follicular unit grafts transplanted directly into the area of previous excisions without reopening. As with follicular unit transplantation procedures in virgin scalps, camouflage sessions should be spaced a minimum of 8-12 months apart. This allows for a better distribution of grafts and permits both the doctor and patient to observe the cosmetic impact of the prior procedure before planning the next.

## Linear Excision

Graft removal via a long, elliptical (oval) excision is useful when grafts are closely packed in a linear arrangement and when the goal is their complete removal, or when it is mandatory that the patient have the removal phase of the repair completed as quickly as possible.

It has been our experience that removing multiple grafts via one long curvilinear excision does not always produce as good a cosmetic result as removing them individually with punches. The reason is that the contraction of the long incision over a curved scalp may cause a slight elevation of one edge of the wound. This tendency may be compounded by the fact that the two edges of the incision have to be angled slightly to match the angle of the hair in the grafts, causing the one angled more acutely to rise up slightly over the other as the wound heals. The multiple small holes created by the punch can often avoid these problems, and heal more consistently with a barely detectable scar. This use of punches must be balanced with the fact that they require more sessions and are not as efficient in removing all of the abnormal grafts as a linear excision.

## Electrolysis

When the underlying scalp is relatively normal in appearance and there is not enough hair in the abnormal grafts for effective re-implantation, removal of the hair alone may be indicated. This situation usually occurs when small micrografts are mistakenly transplanted either too low on the hairline or too far forward in the temples. In this case the underlying skin may be normal and punch excision of the grafts would not only be too aggressive, but the very small punch used might miss a portion of the follicle, resulting in regrowth of the hair. In these situations either electrolysis or laser hair removal would be appropriate to consider.

The success of electrolysis depends upon the operator's ability to insert a fine needle directly into the growth center of the hair follicle. A major limitation to electrolysis in repair is that, because of the scarring, the hair in the grafts tends to be distorted, making accurate needle insertion exceedingly difficult. In addition, the large number of thick coarse hairs makes the procedure slow and tedious and further, electrolysis destroys the hair so that it can't be used again. However, electrolysis may be useful when there are a small number of hairs in the wrong place, and the underlying skin is not significantly scarred.

Any time hair is removed the skin under it becomes more visible. If hair removal is to be used alone, the skin under it must be relatively normal in appearance. Larger grafts universally produce skin changes such as scarring, depigmentation and cobblestoning, so that hair removal alone will not suffice. In these situations, the abnormal skin can be partially removed through excision, improved through procedures such as dermabrasion, or covered with normal appearing follicular units.

## Laser Hair Removal

Laser hair removal is a relatively new technology that offers promise for repair work. As with electrolysis, the hair that is removed cannot be reused and, as with electrolysis, the underlying exposed skin will be left in its previous state. However, the laser has the significant advantage of being effective even when the hair follicles are distorted, since it acts by being absorbed by the pigment in the hair shaft and does not rely on perfectly intact follicular anatomy. Because the laser light is selectively absorbed by melanin, it will work best on those patients with dark hair and light skin, i.e. those who appear most pluggy. It is for these reasons that the laser may be uniquely suited for certain types of repair work.

At the time of this edition, laser hair removal is still classified as "permanent hair reduction." Although the individual treatments are fast, multiple sessions are still required.

## Concept of Camouflage

Camouflage is at the heart of almost all repair procedures. Rarely does one attempt to return the patient to the pre-transplantation state by removing all the problem grafts and rarely can excision and re-implantation alone solve the patient's cosmetic problems. As discussed earlier, camouflage can be performed, with or without prior excision and re-implantation, but if graft removal by any means is planned, it should always be performed before the camouflage is started. There is a natural tendency, when confronted with a repair, to attempt to fill in the gaps between plugs. However, the tendency to "fill in the spaces" between plugs with more plugs, just creates a solid wall of hair and worsens the cosmetic problem. A properly planned camouflage, should not only make the plugs less visible, but also help to redistribute the hair density over a larger area.

Camouflage should not change the actual position of a hairline; that is the job of excision and re-implantation. It is important to emphasize that camouflage changes the hairline's appearance, but not its location. This misconception often makes the patient anxious to bypass the excision part of the procedure, hoping that camouflage alone will solve their problems.

The concept of camouflage is perhaps best explained with the following analogy: If one wants to hide a picket fence, boarding it up will only create a solid wall and make it more obvious. It would be preferable to plant bushes and shrubs on either side of it. The fence would still be in the same position, but not be as visible.

## Establishing the Frontal Hairline

Camouflage is an important repair tool for all parts of the scalp, but using it to help establish a normal appearing hairline is the essence of the repair. It is important to make the frontal hairline as "perfect" as possible, so that the observer's eye will be brought back to the central part of the face rather than searching in other parts of the scalp for additional irregularities. Not only will correcting the hairline improve the patient's frontal presentation, it will allow the hair mass that had been combed forward (to hide the unnatural hairline), to now be available to cover other areas of the scalp. This freedom to redirect the hair via styling is one of the most powerful aspects of a properly planned repair, especially in the face of limited donor reserves.

At the frontal hairline, camouflage is accomplished by creating a "transition zone" between the bald forehead and the abnormal grafts. For reasons discussed in the section, Follicular Unit Transplantation: The Ideal Tool for Repair, the transition zone is best constructed with follicular units, as they will provide excellent camouflage with little additional wounding to the recipient skin and, at the same time, ensure a natural result. Creating a transition zone in a repair differs from creating a frontal hairline in a first-time hair transplant in that a number of additional factors must be taken into account, particularly with regard to depth and the specific arrangement of individual follicular units within the zone. The hair transplant surgeon must have significant experience with repair work to do this properly.

The depth needed for the transition zone will be greatly affected by the degree of plugginess and the patient's hair characteristics. For the same degree of visual plugginess, a greater transition zone will be needed for patients with finer hair or those with dark hair and light skin. Interestingly, coarse hair tends to look the most pluggy, but coarse hair is also the best for the repair, giving patients with the worst appearing transplants a reasonable degree of hope. Occasionally, it may be useful to create a "widow's peak," as a means of breaking up an extremely uniform hairline. This is most effective when the patient had one naturally, but even in other patients, creating a subtle peak may be an extremely effective tool for adding asymmetry to the hairline.

## Angling

Ideally, all transplanted hair should point in the direction that it originally grew. When using plugs was commonplace, improper angling was not only a matter of poor judgment, but was a result of the technical difficulties of placing the large grafts at very acute angles. The angled grafts had a tendency to heal at a different elevation than the natural skin surface due to the contraction of the surrounding connective tissue. As a result, larger grafts often grew more perpendicular to the skin surface than natural hair. Unfortunately, even with the use of smaller grafts, doctors still pay too little attention to the way hair grows in nature.

The simplest approach to improperly angled grafts is removal. In situations where removal is impractical (such as when there are large numbers of small, poorly angled grafts), the doctor faces a dilemma. If one matches the angle of the existing hair, the problem will be compounded, but if the new hair is placed in the proper direction, it may not relate well to the old grafts, creating a v-shaped separation. This problem is resolved by the subtle, but progressive angling of implants away from the improperly placed grafts, so that the new follic-ular units adjacent to the old grafts are almost parallel and the grafts furthest away point in the normal direction.

Correct angling is especially important when covering defects in the crown, either from scalp reduction scars or from old grafts, since the crown is essentially a posterior hairline and the observer looks directly into it. When there are no markings for the natural swirl, a new swirl should be created off-center and angled sharply so that the hair fans out and lies flat, covering the defect.

## Weighting

"Weighting" is one of the most useful tools used to increase the cosmetic impact of a Follicular Unit Transplant, and is an integral part of this procedure. Weighting can be accomplished by either placing the recipient sites closer together in selected regions of the scalp or by using larger follicular units in these areas. In a virgin scalp, both of these techniques are used to "forward weight" the transplant to enhance the patient's frontal view. When using weighting to create central density (such as with a forelock-type distribution), graft sorting alone is the preferred technique, since this will minimize the wounding of the central, less vascular parts of the scalp. Side-weighting is used to enhance a specific styling pattern and is accomplished by using more closely spaced, larger follicular units along the part side of the scalp. It requires a commitment on the part of the patient to continue to use a specific hairstyle. Because of this, side-weighting is rarely considered in the first transplant when the styling preference is not known.

In a repair, these techniques are even more important since the limited donor reserves makes planning around a specific styling pattern critical to achieving the best camouflage. Although the patient's grooming preferences should always be taken into consideration, when there is significant depletion of the donor reserves (and many cosmetic problems) the patient may have few options. The best way of performing the repair must be identified by the physician and explained to the patient in advance. As a general rule, side-to-side grooming with the hair combed diagonally back will give the best over-all coverage. This will enable layering to give fullness to the frontal hairline and allow some of the hair mass to be combed backward to provide indirect coverage to the crown. All things being equal, left-to-right grooming is preferable over right-to-left, since the former is the styling preference of the majority of men and will draw less attention to the transplant. Less commonly, when the major cosmetic defects are in the crown, hair combed straight back will be the most effective.

## The Hockey Stick and Carpet Tacking

In situations where there is a great imbalance in the supply/demand ratio, a more exaggerated form of "side-weighting" called the "hockey-stick" may be useful. This might occur in patients with very low density, when open donor harvesting has severely depleted the donor supply, when plugs are scattered in different cosmetic areas (such as the temples and crown), or when scalp reductions have rendered the patient's donor supply unharvestable (by severely reducing the donor density and/or laxity).

The "hockey stick" is accomplished by placing the majority of the implants along the frontal hairline and along the part side with only lightly scattered follicular units in other areas. This takes advantage of dedicated side-to-side grooming that establishes a frame to the face and adds fullness to the front of the scalp while utilizing a minimal amount of hair in less cosmetically important areas.

The hair used in the more sparse areas are called "tacking hairs." These hairs serve to anchor the hair combed over it from the more densely transplanted areas. Tacking hairs are composed of only 1- and 2-hair follicular units so as to conserve the donor supply and to prevent these rather isolated grafts from looking unnatural themselves. The use of "tacking" hairs helps to keep the longer frontal hairs in place during routine activities, and in the wind.

## Special Cosmetic Problems

- Scalp Reductions
- Severe Scarring and Ridging
- Hair Loss from Face Lifts

### Scalp Reductions

Fortunately, scalp reductions have been performed much less frequently in recent years. Scalp reductions have the undesirable effect of simultaneously causing cosmetic problems and depleting the donor supply needed to correct them. Simply stated, they alter the balance between supply and demand. They increase the demand for hair by producing scars on the top of the head and in the crown that must be camouflaged, alter natural balding patterns, and change hair direction all without significantly adding coverage to the front of the scalp. They diminish supply by decreasing donor density and scalp laxity, thereby minimizing the amount of "movable hair" available for the correction.

These problems can be partially addressed by the "hair conserving" techniques of microscopic dissection. However, after multiple scalp reductions, with even the best techniques, full correction is often not possible. Specific patterns of repair, such as the "hockey stick" described above, used for treating patients who have low donor supply, are especially useful to patients with low donor supply as a result of scalp reductions and scalp lifts.

Another problem created by scalp reductions and scalp lifts is the scar in the crown. This can be camouflaged, but it requires a considerable amount of hair. In addition, the scar tissue limits the amount of hair that can be added in one session, so that multiple sessions are often required. When hair is transplanted directly into the scar, the patient may run the risk of having an abnormal balding pattern as the hair loss progresses. The creation of an off-center swirl, previously discussed, can be used to cover scalp reduction scars without having to place a large amount of hair directly into the scars, and can partially address future balding with its fanning hair pattern.

In general, correcting scalp reductions and their associated defects can be approached in a way similar to the approach used for plugs and a depleted donor supply. That is, to correct the front and one side as much as possible and allow that hair to grow and camouflage problems in the back with either light coverage or tacking hair. Problems specific to poorly executed scalp reductions that can't be camouflaged, such as "dog-ear" deformities, should be addressed prior to the actual camouflage procedure. A "dog-ear" deformity (puckering of excess tissues at the ends of the incision) is caused by the failure of the surgeon to make the length of the incision sufficiently greater than the width or the failure to adequately account for the curvature of the skull. It can be corrected by excision, and the hair in the excised tissue can be dissected into follicular units and re-implanted.

## Severe Scarring and Ridging

Ridging is caused by the body's reaction to the increased volume of tissue associated with larger grafts. Ridging from grafts in the frontal hairline gives the head an elongated rather than rounded frontal appearance that accentuates the defects caused by the grafts themselves.

It is our experience that the growth of grafts in areas of ridging is poor. The area can be improved cosmetically by punching out selected areas of plugs where the ridging is most severe. This will decrease both the plugginess and the tissue volume. It is important to perform a few trial punches to be certain that it heals with less elevation. In some cases, even the trauma of removing the grafts seems to contribute to the hyperfibrotic change. When hyperfibrotic change occurs around slit grafts, especially large ones, deep depressions around the grafts may be seen in conjunction with an exaggerated, tufted appearance of the hair. When this situation is encountered, every attempt should be made to completely remove the grafts.

Once the area of ridging has been improved, it seems to accept grafts better in subsequent sessions, but the growth of newly transplanted hair may still be inconsistent. For this reason, we always try to place follicular units in the normal skin in front of the hyperfibrotic change (if the position of the hairline permits) so that adequate camouflage can be ensured.

## Hair Loss from Facelifts

Hair loss is a common complication of facelifts and brow-lifts, but is rarely anticipated by the patients undergoing these procedures, or by the physicians who perform them. Hair loss due to facelifts and brow-lifts can be due to the following:

1. Destruction of hair from incisions not parallel to the follicles;
2. Destruction of hair from suturing;
3. Destruction of follicles from undermining;
4. Alopecia from excessive skin tension;
5. Alopecia from disruption of the vasculature;
6. Stretched scars devoid of hair;
7. Distortion of the normal hairline from the lift;
8. Decreased density from stretching the scalp;
9. Telogen effluvium from the trauma of the surgery;
10. Telogen effluvium from the anesthesia; and
11. Acceleration of androgenetic alopecia.

It is tempting to perform the hair restoration procedure soon after the face-lift. However, it is preferable to wait at lease one year so that the surgical scars have had a chance to mature, the scalp laxity can return to normal and, most important, that any hair loss from post-surgical effluvium has had time to re-grow.

A problem intrinsic to repairing alopecia from facelift procedures is that the hair may be transplanted into the same spot where future facelift incisions will be placed. If the hair loss from the facelift is not excessive and/or there is a question about long-term donor supply, it may be wise to consider post-poning the repair until after the second face-lift. This is espe-cially important in younger patients where multiple facelifts would be anticipated. If future surgery is anticipated, and if hair loss in the area surrounding the surgical incisions is the main problem (rather than the scars themselves), one may place hair only in the surrounding areas of thinning and not in the actual scar. Another way to circumvent this problem is to avoid "aggressive" lifts or postpone aspects of the procedure that are more likely to result in hair loss, such as a brow lift. A second problem inherent in facelifts is that when the deci-sion is made to perform the procedure, the signs of androgenic alopecia may not yet be present (or if present, not taken into adequate consideration). In a patient with no apparent hair loss, potential androgenetic alopecia may be suspected from a positive family history or the presence of miniaturization greater than 20% in the front or top of the scalp.

When hair loss follows facelifts, the entire frontal hairline extending down to the sideburn area often needs to be restored. In female patients, it is important to maintain the rounded female hairline. The hair direction in women is usu-ally more varied than the predominately forward direction of the average male hairline. The female hairline is often char-acterized by "licks" and "peaks" and these should be restored to achieve the optimum results. Especially with brow lifts, there may be broad areas of thinning both anterior and poste-rior to the coronal incision. These regions should be filled with follicular units as closely spaced as the physician can comfortably manage, since transplanted hair, when compared with the more dense hair directly behind it, will generally appear too thin. Once the first few millimeters of the hairline have been transplanted with smaller units, the largest follicular units should be used to achieve the greatest frontal density possible. In spite of this, it may still take several procedures to achieve satisfactory density.

In contrast to men, many women have fine, vellus hairs at their frontal hairline. Since donor hair is generally harvested from the mid-portion of the permanent zone, the diameter of this hair may be too great for the frontal hairline or temples. If the match is not right (a situation that is more often seen in women with darker, coarse hair) finer hair should be used. Using the fine hair lower down on the posterior scalp or behind the ears is not recommended for this purpose. As will be explained in the next section, scars placed below the occipital ridge will tend to stretch, and those behind the ear may interfere with further facelifts. The preferred method of generating finer hair is to remove all or part of a terminal hair's bulb prior to implantation.

## Donor Area Repair

Prior to undertaking a scar revision in the donor area, it is important to take a careful history and find out specifically what, if anything went wrong with the previous surgeries. It is presumptuous to think that just because a patient has scarring, the next procedure will make it better. The first thing that the surgeon should do is to carefully review the surgical history and, if possible, speak with the original surgeon to see if there are any techniques that could be improved upon or identifiable problems that could have been avoided.

The cause of an unacceptable scar may have been due to poor healing intrinsic to the patient, such as the tendency to form keloids. It may have been caused by a genetic or drug induced bleeding problem, or a medication that interfered with healing. Scarring may have been due to a complication such as a post-operative infection or simply from the patient not following post-op instructions by performing strenuous exercise, or resuming smoking too soon after the surgery.

A depleted donor supply is the major limitation to a successful repair. The inability to harvest additional hair is caused by two main factors. The first is the physical limit set by low donor density and poor scalp mobility. In the face of low donor density, a larger strip must be harvested to obtain an adequate amount of hair. A tight scalp, however, limits the size of the strip that can be removed. After multiple procedures, the surgeon begins to reach a point of diminishing returns, where trying to harvest additional hair is no longer worth the risk of a possible widened scar. Every hair transplant procedure simultaneously decreases donor density and scalp laxity, but poorly executed surgery does this to a greater degree and decreases the supply without making proportionate cosmetic improvements in the recipient scalp.

The second factor is the visibility of the donor scars themselves. Once the donor scars are to the point of near visibility, the ability to harvest additional hair is severely limited. An important point to keep in mind in judging how much additional hair is available is that coverage of donor scarring is more closely related to the amount of donor hair present, than to the degree of scarring. Therefore, any process that removes hair, along with the scar, will run the risk of making the donor scar more visible, not less. When scar and hair are both removed, the closure will further stretch the scalp and decrease the density of the remaining hair. This may prevent it from covering other scars that have not been excised. It may also thin out the appearance of the donor fringe to an unacceptable degree.

## Excisional Repair

Excisional repair should be considered when scarring is localized and the cosmetic benefit from its removal will be more than offset by the decreased density of the surrounding hair. Because of the importance of the surrounding area for camouflage, success in decreasing the size of an existing scar depends as much upon the choice of the scar as upon the actual surgical technique used to repair it.

There are a number of surgical techniques that have the tendency to produce poor donor scars. An understanding of how these may contribute to poor wound healing helps to explain the appropriate approach for their repair. The more common problems include:

- Deep donor incisions
- Wide donor strips
- Suturing with large bites
- Non-contour incisions
- Donor incisions placed too low
- Donor incisions placed too high

## Deep Donor Incisions

The fascia acts as a structural support to the healing wound. When this support has been injured, the risk of having a widened scar is greatly increased. The use of copious amounts of anesthetic fluid infiltrated directly into the subcutaneous fat will elevate the scalp and increase the distance from the base of the follicles to the fascia. This is probably the single best way to keep the wound superficial. When the wound is superficial, then the donor strip may be removed with the least amount of harm to the fascia.

When proper superficial harvesting of the donor strip is performed, and there is no undue tension on the wound, a layered closure is rarely, if ever, needed. There is no concern that the deeper sutures will impinge on follicles, and there is no need to suture the fascia, as it is already intact. In contrast, with a repair a meticulous layered closure is sometimes important because there is often significant wound tension and the sutured scar tissue regains its wound strength more slowly than normal hair-bearing scalp.

## Wide Donor Strips

In the era of megasessions, the problem of taking too wide a donor strip is an increasingly common problem. A wide strip places unnecessary tension on the donor closure and leads to a widened scar. When larger sessions are appropriate, and the scalp does not have high mobility, the surgeon should consider a longer incision rather than a wider one.

If a wide initial incision is identified as the likely cause of a widened scar, we suggest waiting at least 8 months so that the scar may mature and the scalp laxity return. On re-excision, it is advisable to make the new strip at least 3-6mm (or more) narrower than the previous one. When a tight closure is the cause of a widened scar, one should generally not attempt to remove the entire width of the old scar since this invariably leads to a reoccurrence, or worsening, of the old scar. However, the new excision can extend into one hair-bearing edge. In other situations, when adequate laxity is present, removing the entire scar width may be beneficial. When two hair-bearing areas are placed next to each other, the healing seems to be improved.

## Suturing with Large Bites

When suturing with large bites, a significant amount of hair-bearing scalp is incorporated within the sutures. Especially with a running stitch suture, any post-op edema or tension in the donor area will tend to limit the blood supply of the entrapped tissue and may result in permanent hair loss. In addition, if there is any tension on the wound, the mechanical pressure of the sutures alone can cause hair loss. In the repair, horizontal mattress sutures may be used to reduce wound tension followed by the use of small bites very close to the wound edge in the superficial closure.

## Non-Contour Incisions

Incisions that do not follow the natural curved contour of

the scalp tend to heal with wider scars than those that follow the contour of the skull. When a re-excision is planned, it is important to have the new excision follow the natural curvature of the skull, regardless of the linearity of the original excision and regardless of whether the new excision completely encompasses the old one. The focus should be on reducing the size of the original scar and changing its direction, rather than eliminating it totally.

### Donor Incisions Placed too Low

Of the various factors contributing to a widened donor scar, the most problematic with respect to the repair is having placed the initial incision too low on the posterior scalp. Some doctors feel that hair lower down on the scalp is a good source of fine hair, but it has been our experience that this hair may not be permanent and that this practice is associated with too great a risk of unacceptable scarring. Incisions that lie too low on the back of the scalp will be affected by the muscle movement directly below them and have a much greater tendency to stretch.

It has been our experience that even the conservative re-excision of a widened scar that is located in the inferior portion of the occipital scalp carries a significant risk of healing with an even wider scar. Scars in this area should not be re-excised and, if additional transplants are performed, hair should be harvested from an incision made above it, leaving a thin zone of hair separating the upper and lower incisions. Instead of attempting to remove the scar, its appearance may be more consistently improved by the addition of small amounts of hair to the area, with far less risk.

### Donor Incisions Placed too High

When a donor incision has been placed too high, it is best left untreated unless the scar is wide and poor surgical technique has been identified as the cause. Often, the surgeon making the poor judgment in placing the wound too high has done an equally poor job in the closure, so that there is a reasonable chance the scar may be improved upon with better techniques. As with other scars, however, one should generally attempt to lessen or improve the configuration, rather than completely remove the scar.

The temptation to add hair into the scar should be resisted, since progressive balding would isolate the hair-bearing scar and present new cosmetic problems demanding additional hair. An exception to this would be placing hair into the lower portion of a vertical scalp reduction scar that dips way down into the permanent donor area.

## Implantation of Hair

When a localized area of a donor scar is cosmetically bothersome, its excision is impractical, and there is easily accessible donor hair in other areas, it sometimes will benefit the patient to place hair directly into the widened donor scar. Two-hair follicular units are the most useful for this purpose and should be inserted at very acute angles. Only a small amount of hair is usually needed to soften the appearance of a scar and dedicating too much hair for this purpose is unnecessary and wasteful.

## A Final Word on Repair

The physician attempting a repair faces a set of challenges quite different from operating on a virgin scalp. The patient frequently has dramatic cosmetic defects, a severely limited donor supply and, too often, hopelessness at the prospect of looking normal again. In reparative surgery, the support of the physician is essential, the judicious use of every graft is critical, and setting priorities in the restorative process becomes as important as the surgical technique itself.

# 21

## CHOOSING YOUR DOCTOR

Technically perfect results can fail to live up to the client's expectations if there was a failure of communication between the client and the physician. Perfection in the art of hair restoration is a judgment call that can only be determined by the satisfaction of the patient. It is crucial that the potential client weigh the advantages and disadvantages of each medical group. In selecting one's doctor, the most important decision factors should be tied to the surgeon's expertise and the value of the relationship between the physician and the patient.

A potential client should be wary of marketing techniques that are common to the promotion of expensive services and products. Such sales aides include fancy brochures, videos, and slick, high-pressure sales techniques. Sometimes, video presentations are used to demonstrate a physician's notoriety on talk shows. Video imaging techniques often show an unrealistic presentation of a potential outcome. These techniques are used to divert the attention of the potential customer from the basic physician/patient relationship. Invest the time to know your doctor, his standards, and his approach to your questions. The amount of time the doctor is willing to spend with you should be an important factor in your judgment of his or her true interest in your satisfaction. No matter how eager you may be to get started, remember that a hair restoration procedure is permanent. Do not rush your decision on selecting a physician; do your homework carefully. A good decision today is a good decision tomorrow.

Male Pattern Baldness is a process that occurs in cycles over time. The client has lost hair in the past and will lose additional hair in the future. The assessment of a patient's needs to restore his hairline or to cover a bald spot must include a plan to cover his likely future needs. This requires a realistic estimate of what those needs are likely to be. The doctor should inform his or her patient of probable future hair loss and explain that while hair loss is progressive, it is cyclical with alternating periods of slow and rapid hair loss.

## Is Your Doctor Board Certified?

"Board Certified" means the doctor has had residency training and passed an oral and written examination in a certain specialty. In general, doctors who have received specialty surgical training perform surgical procedures more competently than other doctors. Some physicians have developed considerable expertise in hair restoration without having had specialty training in any field. It is a good idea to discuss the experiences that they feel make them qualified to work in this field.

General training in hair transplantation is found in dermatology residency programs throughout the world (less often in plastic surgery or cosmetic surgery training programs), but these programs often teach outdated, traditional hair transplant techniques. Most hair transplant surgeons pick up their techniques from books, articles, medical meetings on the subject, or from a modified "apprenticeship" programs. To date, there are no watchdog committees, no specialty certifications available, and essentially no way for a prospective patient to verify the competence of his or her physician through a credentialing process. Educational societies are forming and will eventually evolve into certification organizations. The need for formal certification is critical to the proper growth of this specialty. Currently, a prospective surgical candidate must rely on his or her own diligence to confirm a physician's claim of competence the hair transplant field.

## Experience

Ask the doctor how much experience he or she has had in performing hair transplant surgery and why he or she feels qualified to do this type of work.

NHI trains and certifies all its affiliated physicians. They are schooled in the principles and surgical techniques of hair transplantation, even if they have prior hair transplantation experience. Before allowing new physicians to see patients under NHI's endorsement, the physicians are carefully observed. By choosing a NHI physician, you gain the benefit of high standards and uniformity of process.

NHI backs the quality and skills of its doctors. Their skills meet one standard. Their judgments in hairline design and the quality of their work is uniform. The doctors selected for affiliation with the New Hair Institute have committed themselves to a high standard of care and have proven themselves many times. Each affiliated doctor is re-certified yearly.

## Type of Practice

Does the doctor specialize in hair transplant procedures? Hair transplantation should be a major focus of the doctor's practice.

## Time

Does the doctor spend enough time with you during the consultation? It takes time for a complete evaluation, discussion and to understand one's needs and expectations. Evaluate the time spent with the doctor one on one in addition to time spent with a knowledgeable member of the doctor's staff.

## Congeniality

You will probably have to visit the doctor more than once; it is easier if you like the doctor and if you feel safe and secure with him or her. The relationship can be difficult or impossible to establish if either one does not like the other.

## Trust

Trust and honesty are crucial elements of the doctor/patient relationship. If there is no trust, the relationship is unsound. A poor relationship can produce results that are not satisfactory. Choose a doctor who you feel is honest and who you can trust. Although this type of surgery is not a life or death affair, the whole world will be able to see the results.

## Speak With the Doctor and Examine His or Her Patients

The best way to choose a doctor is to speak with and, if possible, examine one or more of the doctor's patients. A physician with a successful practice can usually ask some patients to share their results with prospective newcomers. Most doctors have one or two patients who are so satisfied that they are willing to speak with other prospective patients on a routine basis. If the doctor is willing to offer this option, it will give prospective patients the opportunity to see the quality of the work performed and it should add comfort to the doctor/patient relationship.

When you meet a patient, examine his hair. If the patient will not let you touch his hair, this should alert you to some abnormality he is conscious about or covering up. If that should occur, confront the issue directly. Look at the skin at scalp level. Is it pitted? Are there skin distortions that look like a cobblestoned street? Does the hair sprout from the scalp like a fern? Would you be satisfied with that appearance if your hair loss were equal to his? Ask about the technical details of the procedure. Ask how much discomfort he had. Compare his situation and appearance with your own.

Examine the area where the donor hair was taken, usually on the back and/or sides of the head. Is it badly scarred? Is it noticeable? Is there more than one scar? If the person had scalp reductions or flaps, ask how the hair looks when not groomed. Does it cause a problem when he sweats, swims, plays tennis, or jogs? Does he have scars that are difficult to hide?

Ask the patient whether he would go through the procedure again. Is he satisfied? Were his expectations met? Does he have confidence in the doctor? Why did he select that particular doctor? Did he participate in the decision process? Did the doctor's estimates of the work reflect the reality of the work? Did the patient you interviewed (in person or by phone) seem believable?

One or two such interviews should give you all the information you need. The best research for any product or service is accomplished by talking with a knowledgeable customer. Do not set unrealistic demands upon the doctor by asking him to arrange interviews with a patient who has your exact hair color, hair characteristics, extent of hair loss, and the like. If you do this, you will never find a doctor who will pass your test.

If the doctor fails to pay attention to your needs, you should be on the alert. Is this doctor really the proper one for you? Tell your doctor about any uneasiness you feel. Give the doctor a chance to answer your questions and address your problems directly. Remember a good decision today is a good decision tomorrow! Do not let anyone pressure you into making a decision you may regret for the rest of your life! Be wary of doctor's offices that call you repeatedly to intimidate or rush you into going forward. Do not accept a doctor who pushes you into a decision. Do not accept a physician substitute in what must be a very personal doctor/patient relationship. Salesmen (or the like) are paid to sell you on a purchase. This is a decision to undergo a surgical procedure and pressure sales play no role with ethical practitioners.

## Skill of Each Team Member

A happy, comfortable environment is critical to the efficiency and productivity of each participant, but efficiency and productivity alone do not produce quality work. It is in the preparation and placement of the grafts that the success of the transplant is determined. NHI has seen many patients who have had work performed elsewhere and the transplants never grew or did not yield the full amount of viable hair follicles expected. One can count the number of hairs in the larger grafts that survive, and by knowing or guessing their original size; one can estimate the survival rate of the hair follicles. Death of hair follicles may reflect improper handling procedures during the critical process of graft preparation or poor technique when harvesting the grafts from the donor area.

## Standards of Practice

Hair transplantation requires unusually high ethical standards. Generally, all doctors subscribe to the principle "above all do no harm". They take this to mean: do not inflict physical pain or harm upon a patient. However, doctors who are familiar with the short view of a usual medical or surgical treatment may not adjust well to the long-term view of a hair transplantation process. If a doctor does something wrong in a typical surgery for example, problems are usually quick to appear, so that the learning process is fast.

In hair transplantation, the results of the surgery may not be significant until 8 months after a procedure, and full benefits may not be achieved for a year or two. In traditional hair transplantation, (many surgeries spaced months apart), the process may take years. For the large sessions of smaller grafts, the learning cycle will be shorter, as the process is significantly contracted from beginning to end.

It is too easy for a physician to conclude that hair transplant surgery is a simple procedure that any trained, competent technician should be able to do. This is far from the truth.

There has been a high demand for hair transplant services, but there are a limited number of reputable surgeons. These factors produce high prices as well as many opportunities for second-class quality. Too often, patients do not demand accountability from their doctors. This is apparent in the way the industry goes about its business today. Many doctors employ salesmen to protect themselves from patients and their expectations. Beware of language devised to enhance the doctor's influence. Doctors who claim to have invented or originated a whatever-a-graft or a what-a-plasty generally mean that they devised the name with the purpose of confusing, rather than educating, the patient. The use of Latin sounding names (galia, mono, varia, etc.) may also indicate such intentions.

NHI is not against using names that serve an educational or descriptive purpose, but physicians who use such terms should define them and use them in a context that enhances the communication process. Our use of "Fast Track", for example, was designed to enhance the understanding of the time commitment in the hair transplantation process.

Beware of an unbalanced focus upon special glues, the use of dilators (finishing nails which hold your graft holes open prior to graft insertion), or bandaging techniques. In addition, some doctors actually make it a point to be photographed with a political figure, a famous actor, etc., in order to imply positive endorsement. True indications of value are teaching positions, research in the field, or publication of books and articles. The publication of written material in approved, peer-reviewed journals reflects contributions to the field of hair restoration that have merit based upon content. Watch out for organizations that confuse facts, present their services like used car dealerships, harass you with persistent phone calls under the guise of following up on your initial contact, and similar tactics. The patient who expresses an urgent need to get hair back at any cost is the best test of the ethical standards of the hair restoration doctor. The doctor should be responsible for setting proper expectations, communicating fully about the process, and insulating the prospective patient from the commercial selling process. The doctor should slow down the decision process if the patient appears to be making an impetuous decision.

Balding is not sudden; it takes time to evolve. Restoring hair should be a thoughtful process: it is not an emergency. Do not rush forward and make a mistake by starting something you are not willing or able to complete. Do your homework. Meet and view patients with results that you feel meet your standard of quality. Plan your budget carefully. Get to know your doctor and be sure he is a competent, caring and ethical.

## The Aesthetic Aspect

The surgeon must understand the nuances in integrating the various characteristics of hair, how it grows, its color and contrast to the skin, and the ethnic attributes of the patient, to blend them in a natural-looking way. The surgeon must also meet the objectives of the patient. This is not as easy as it sounds. It requires spending time with each patient, to understand what the patient wants to achieve. The surgeon should not dictate rules by which the patient must abide; it is not the doctor who will live with the appearance created by the surgery for the rest of his or her life. Too many surgeons dictate where the hairline should be placed or where they place the hair they move, when the patient's opinions should play a significant role in these decisions.

Most frequently, the hair restoration surgeon is not able to ascertain just how to balance the long-term process of hair loss with the short-term goals of the patient. The patient wants to believe that his short-term goal, when met, is compatible with a normal long-term appearance. Selling short-term goals without regard to the long-term outcome is irresponsible and one of the most common problems with this industry. The potential conflict of interest of a less than honorable doctor may precipitate too much surgery and too much expense to the patient. It is all too easy to promise and deliver the patient's short-term needs by setting him up to look like a freak in the long-term as his hair loss progresses to its natural inherited conclusion.

Take great care in analyzing the aesthetic capabilities of the surgeon you choose, as hair transplantation is permanent. A hairline placed too low, will be too low for the life of the patient and a low hairline cannot be moved higher.

Hair loss is a lifetime process and the hair transplant surgeon starts mid-process with an uncertain and unpredictable hair loss pattern. It is critical that any additional hair transplants fit into a "master plan" considering a worst-case scenario. After the surgeon finishes the restoration, the hair loss of the patient does not miraculously stop. It continues through its natural course, one that may be different from what anyone expected. The long-term nature of hair loss means that the work performed must be intrinsically flexible in its design and capable of appearing natural in the context of a worst-case hair loss pattern, if that should develop.

It is important that each procedure stand on its own, as much as possible. This means that, after having one procedure, the patient should be able to stop if he wishes. If not, he should be informed of the consequences of further hair loss as part of the informed consent process. Great care must be taken to understand the incremental value of each procedure. Ask if one procedure will require more procedures. In traditional transplants, stopping with less than the required number of procedures will create a visibly obvious "half-done" job. Everyone will be able to see a deformity appearing as a "toothbrush" hairline.

NHI has rarely seen a completed hair transplant patient with advanced balding using the older transplant approach. Most people with traditional hair transplants stop before they finish. They may just get fed up with the never-ending process, they may run out of money, run out of hair, or they may just give up on what seems to be an unattainable goal. This does not happen when the Fast Track® is performed on an informed patient using Follicular Grafts.

## Young Men: Attention!

All too often, a 25 year-old says: "I don't care what I look like when I'm 50, just give me hair now." This type of comment is a red flag indicating unrealistic expectations and potential lack of foresight. Every 50-year-old man we've ever met still cares what he looks like! Bad planning and poor design are the worst enemies of the young candidate who will pay for any promise, real or imaginary, for the return of the hair he can never really get back.

## The Technical Aspect

The hair transplant surgeon must have high aesthetic standards and be skilled in sophisticated surgical techniques. Transplantation of a large number of grafts in a single session can be a long procedure for the patient and arduous work for the medical team. A focus upon both the patient's needs and the surgical team's experience is critical. Safety and comfort of the patient must be central to the entire approach.

Hair restoration procedures have evolved significantly over the past decade. Hundreds of thousands of patients have had various types of hair restoration procedures performed with results ranging from near perfection to dismal. Naiveté runs rampant in the medical community, even among the physicians who specialize in hair transplants. Many hair transplant physicians are afraid to follow up with their patients because of a fear of the patient's results. In addition, we have seen hair transplant specialists who have actually performed the procedure on members of their own staffs or had the procedures performed on themselves with substandard results. As a potential patient, if you make this type of observation, you should reassess any proposed procedure. In this field, what you see is what you get.

## The Medical Group's Style and Presentation

The field of hair transplantation is overrun with misinformation. Unsubstantiated claims in the media often delude potential patients. Some large medical groups run aggressive advertising campaigns that create an image of unrealistic results using expensive, well-designed brochures to drive the message home. Prospective clients are frequently delivered into the hands of high-pressure salesmen working for such clinics. Claims that improperly represent that a complete hair restoration is reasonable in men who have lost 75% of their hair (Norwood Class 7 patients) are all too frequent. The decision to undergo such a procedure is too often made under pressure, and reality is often glossed over by unscrupulous entrepreneurs or naive physicians who practice an art form they do not really understand. For the hair transplant patients who had their work before the introduction of the smaller graft, the actual number of dissatisfied patients may be higher. With the introduction of the smaller graft and a significant reduction of the pluggy look, the number of dissatisfied patients has decreased substantially. In these smaller graft patients, the main cause of dissatisfaction usually results from an inadequate amount of work, or the setting of unrealistic expectations, not necessarily an abnormal appearing result.

Lack of adequate, informed consent runs rampant in this field. As a result, a language has developed with a special jargon to describe the outcome with metaphors such as "the toothbrush look," "doll's head look," and the "pluggy look." These are all terms, used to describe the problems faced by many of the patients who had extensive hair restoration procedures before the widespread use of the smaller graft.

The damage of a poor hair transplant procedure goes far beyond what is visible. Psychological damage can be extensive and social problems are all too frequent. Some patients become reclusive; they live in restricted worlds, refusing to go into public or do so only under controlled conditions. For a person sensitive to his appearance, meeting new people or going to a social function can become an ordeal. If social visibility is necessary in the person's occupation, his career can be destroyed. Personal relationships are often affected. Self-consciousness and insecurity can lead to depression.

Many victims of substandard hair restoration surgical procedures find solace in hairpieces and toupees; the very thing they tried to avoid in the first place. The decision to acquire a toupee may be the only way to achieve some degree of normalcy. Some victims go from doctor to doctor undergoing more surgical procedures. Each new doctor is seen as another messiah, but the chance of finding miracles diminishes as each new procedure is added.

# 22

## WHEN TO BE SUSPICIOUS

Some dishonest doctors suggest that you try a few hair transplant grafts to see if you like them. They may suggest that a few grafts do not commit you to a complete course. This is not true. Like it or not, as you progress in your hair loss process, a small number of grafts are likely to create a medical oddity at some point in the future. The following is a list of rules to follow when looking for a hair transplant physician:

- Avoid doctors who use salesmen or non-medical people with no experience or formal training.

- Avoid doctors who use promotions or pressure you into making a decision.

- Avoid doctors who do not spend enough time to listen to your needs and understand your goals.

- Avoid doctors who quote you unrealistically low or high amounts of work, time, or money.

- Avoid doctors who tell you that their patients will not show off their results.

- Avoid doctors or salesman who tell you only good stories. Are they trying to hide something? Do they have the rapport with their patients that they claim? There are always down sides to any surgical procedure and these must be part of the information relayed to you.

Are your doctor and his staff honest and forthright about the potential downside? Proper informed consent is required by law.

- Avoid doctors who specialize in minigrafts and recommend performing monthly sessions. If subsequent transplants are performed before the previously transplanted hair grows, the previous grafts may not be identified and could be damaged.

Until recently, anyone trying to find accurate information about hair replacement has faced a confusing and difficult task. Much of the literature about various hair restoration options aimed to sell you something. Deliberately confusing advertising from wig salesmen, surgeons experimenting with new techniques, and charlatans who scrub clogged pores to cure balding, were some of the obstacles one had to deal with. There is often a fine line between ignorance and incompetence in the hair restoration field, so the buyer of these services must exercise careful judgment when reviewing the material.

Doctors or scientists usually announce advances in medicine to their peers in medical or scientific journals. The public finds out about them later via mass media. This has not always been the case with hair restoration advances, as promotions by physicians often create false impressions of what is possible in terms of treatment.

Sophisticated techniques for hair restoration that achieve truly natural-looking results have only become available relatively recently. Unfortunately, many doctors practicing hair restoration are unaware of these advances. Widespread ignorance prevails throughout the medical profession on the subject of hair. Hair transplantation, as developed in the late 1950s, is still practiced with the large-graft techniques that produce a pluggy or patchy look.

In any field, advertising is an important way to educate the public, especially in the early phase of an industry's growth. Hair restoration physicians have used advertising for years. Because of the marketing in the late 1990's of Rogaine by Upjohn Company and Propecia by Merck, consumer awareness has reached a new peak. Many people want their hair back, as sales figures for Rogaine indicate. Good specialists in any field are hard to find, and understanding what your real options are can be very confusing. In surgical solutions, a mistake with the wrong hair restoration procedure or the wrong doctor can be a mistake for life. The problem that confronts prospective buyers is how to recognize a doctor's ability, honesty, and his or her standards in a specialized field where exaggerated claims abound.

Beware of slick brochures and claims that appear outstanding on the surface. Mentally subtract the glitz, and see if the written material has merit without the glossy pictures. Be dubious when literature displays beautiful women inappropriately. Do some research and see if the claims are accurate. If a brochure claims to condemn salesmen in the early presentation of the subject material, see if the medical group practices what they preach. Do they use salesmen as a primary advertising tactic? If the medical group invites you to meet with a doctor, do you actually get to meet with a doctor? Is the service personalized? Do patients have easy access to the physician after his fees are paid?

# 23

## COMMON FALLACIES IN HAIR TRANSPLANTATION

The following sections address some fallacies commonly disseminated by hair transplant surgeons still using the older techniques.

### Fallacy #1
### A large number of small grafts cannot get the needed blood supply to grow properly.

*Explanation:*
Since the scalp has one of the richest blood supplies of any region of the body, and its blood supply is anastomotic (comes from many directions and is all interconnected), it can easily support large numbers of grafts, provided that the wounds made in the recipient site are very small. The great advantage of Follicular Unit Transplantation is that the grafts are small enough to fit into very tiny recipient sites. Those who make these comments usually have little experience with using small grafts and do not understand the anatomy of the scalp's blood flow and graft oxygenation. The main issue is one of oxygen diffusion. Since oxygen must diffuse into the center of the newly transplanted graft, very large grafts will be oxygen-deprived in their center. This has been shown repeatedly by observing the phenomenon called doughnutting, the loss of hair follicles in the center of larger grafts. This phenomenon is noted in larger grafts, but does not occur in follicular unit

grafts since the distance that oxygen must travel to reach the center of the graft is so short.

## Fallacy #2
### Large grafts produce a better, denser transplant than smaller grafts.

*Explanation:*

The density of a given area is determined by the total amount of hair transplanted, not by the size of the grafts. Larger grafts do not ultimately give you more hair; rather, they produce an unnatural look. The highest quality hair transplants require fine instruments and large numbers of delicate, small grafts. These grafts must be distributed in a way that balances the patient's individual facial features and hair characteristics. Large grafts do not offer sufficient flexibility to allow this "customizing," and they weight the transplanted area out of proportion to the rest of the scalp.

## Fallacy #3
### Larger grafts can produce a denser hairline than smaller grafts

*Explanation:*

While this statement is literally true, it represents a misunderstanding of the true aim of a hair transplant. The goal should not be to establish a dense, abrupt hairline, but rather to create a natural-looking hairline. A very dense hairline is not appropriate for most people as they age, just as a very flat hairline is not appropriate. This is especially true for someone who has less hair due to thinning or balding. It is up to the surgeon to    balance density and naturalness    to give his patient the best possible appearance. A dense frontal hairline made with larger grafts will never look as natural as a properly designed hairline using fine delicate grafts. The density of the transplanted area should always be appropriate for the long-term goals of the individual.

## Fallacy #4
### "Try a few grafts and see if hair transplantation is for you."

*Explanation:*

This statement is one of the most disturbing comments made by a doctor. The "try a few" mentality is, in our opinion, tantamount to medical malpractice, as it does not fully inform the patient of the potential problems of starting a process that he or she may not wish to complete.

## Fallacy #5
### With a young balding man, the doctor rubs the hair in the back and sides of his head and announces: "You have plenty of hair for a transplant."

*Explanation:*

Each one of us is born with a different, but finite, quantity of hair. New hair cannot be created. Scientific measurements (of hair density), such as densitometry, provide the surgeon with much greater accuracy than subjective assessments when estimating the total supply of permanent hair. The importance of accurately estimating the total donor reserves for proper long-term planning cannot be over emphasized. Beware of any doctor who says that you are a great candidate for a transplant before he spends the time to carefully examine you.

## Fallacy #6
### By cutting out some of the bald area in the back, scalp reductions save hair for future loss in the front.

*Explanation:*

Such statements reflect an unacceptable lack of knowledge. Hair is a limited resource that is depleted regardless of how it is moved. A scalp reduction is not a magical process (as it is often portrayed). It moves hair to the front of the scalp at the expense of the back. With a scalp reduction, the hair in the donor area is thinned considerably, and the scalp's laxity (looseness) is decreased as the scalp is stretched to cover new area. This means that when the frontal hair is lost, the surgeon may not be able to harvest the quantity of hair needed to meet the patient's needs, as the hair supply might run out before the completion of surgery.

As most people want to frame their faces, the frontal restoration usually takes precedence over the crown for hair redistribution purposes. If the crown is treated first, the surgeon must be certain from the very start that the way the hair is distributed leaves enough hair in reserve to cover the remainder of the balding scalp. Scalp reductions, by addressing the crown first, significantly compromise this principle. In addition, scalp reductions can cause problems such as scarring, a thinned scalp, altered hair direction, and a host of other unwanted effects, that become more and more difficult to deal with as the patient's baldness progresses.

## Fallacy #7
### Removing large amounts of donor hair is unsafe.

*Explanation:*

The judgment of an experienced surgeon will insure that the amount of hair that is harvested from the donor area is safe and appropriate. If follicular dissection is performed carefully using microscopes, the amount of hair needed for the average large session is well within the safe limits of transplantation. The amount of moveable donor hair reflects the size of the donor area, the scalp's looseness, the number of hairs per square inch, and the amount of scarring (if any) from previous surgeries. These factors must be considered before the surgical procedure, ideally during the patient's initial evaluation.

## Fallacy #8
## With new laser technology, recipient sites can be made without injury to the transplanted area.

*Explanation:*

Lasers were introduced to hair transplantation to produce slits that were supposed to look better than punch holes, and to remove tissue to accommodate large grafts. The exclusive use of follicular units eliminates the need for lasers since the small grafts fit into very tiny micro-slits that can be created without removing tissue. Regardless of how precise the laser beam, or how small the zone of thermal burn around the wound that the laser produces, the laser still makes a hole or slit by destroying and removing tissue. This is essentially the same type of wound produced by the cold steel punches of the early days of hair transplantation. Lasers will always produce more injury to the recipient area than a micro-slit that does not remove tissue.

# 24

# A FINAL NOTE

In this book, we have presented a detailed overview of hair loss and its treatment. We have tried to offer a clear explanation of the various options available to men and women who are experiencing hair loss. The most common and rational options concerning medications, surgery, and hair systems have been discussed. Only by becoming an informed consumer can you make the right decision for yourself. The following points are important to remember:

- Hair loss starts at varying ages. Some individuals become bald by their 20's, or balding can slowly progress throughout adult life. Although you may sense that you are losing hair by simple observation, your physician can make a specific diagnosis of hair loss.

- There are many options for hair replacement today, from medications to hairpieces to surgical procedures. Be sure that you understand both the advantages and the risks before you begin any course of treatment.

- The FDA approved medications, finasteride and minoxidil, can significantly delay the progression of hairloss and reverse early thinning. There are many more unproven remedies on the market. A knowledgeable doctor is the best source of information about these options.

- Make sure that when you go to see a physician for

your hair loss problems you see the actual doctor. Do not settle for a salesman in a white coat.

- Be certain your doctor understands your goals, needs, and expectations. Be certain that he or she performs only state-of-the-art surgical techniques or can refer you to a physician who does.

- Once popular procedures, such as scalp reduction and flaps, have an unacceptable rate of problems and are no longer used by most hair restoration surgeons. Some newly "hyped" procedures such as laser hair transplantation, may also cause more harm than good, and are not recommended by most physicians.

- Commonly practiced techniques, such as mini-micro-grafting, although relatively quick and easy to perform, rely on a multi-bladed knife to remove the donor tissue and can cause excessive hair wastage and less than natural results.

- Only techniques using single strip harvesting and stereo-microscopic dissection can insure that the donor supply is used efficiently and without waste, and only Follicular Unit Transplantation can insure natural results.

- The physicians of the New Hair Institute first published an article discussing Follicular Unit Transplantation in 1995. This procedure has now become the "gold standard" of surgical hair restoration. To be performed properly, Follicular Unit requires a surgeon who understands both the artistic and technical complexities of transplanting large numbers of very small grafts, a surgical team specifically trained in the stereo-microscopic dissection of follicular units, and facilities that are specifically equipped to perform this labor intensive, exacting procedure.

- Hair transplantation is moderately expensive but, in the long run, can be far less costly than other treatments. Transplanted hair behaves like the original hair. It grows and must be cut and styled like normal hair. If transplantation is performed properly, your transplant ed hair can look perfectly normal and last a lifetime.

We hope that the information provided in this text has been helpful and we wish you luck in your search for a hair loss solution that will be right for you.

# SELECTED REFERENCES

1.  Bernstein RM, Rassman WR, Szaniawski W, Halperin A. Follicular Transplantation. Intl J Aesthetic Restorative Surg 1995; 3:119-132.

2.  Bernstein RM: Are scalp reductions still indicated? Hair Transplant Forum Intl 1996; 6(3):12-13.

3.  Bernstein RM, Rassman WR. Laser hair transplantation: is it really state of the art? Lasers in Surgery and Medicine 1996; 19:233-235.

4.  Bernstein RM, Rassman WR. What is delayed growth? Hair Transplant Forum Intl 1997; 7(2):22.

5.  Bernstein RM, Rassman WR. Follicular transplantation: patient evaluation and surgical planning. Dermatol Surg 1997; 23:771-784.

6.  Bernstein RM, Rassman WR. The aesthetics of follicular transplantation. Dermatol Surg 1997; 23:785-799.

7.  Bernstein RM. Measurements in hair restoration. Hair Transplant Forum Intl. 1998; 8(1):27.

8.  Bernstein RM. Commentary on the origin of follicular unit transplantation. Dermatol Surg 1998; 24(8):929-932.

9.  Rassman WR, Bernstein RM. Rapid Fire Hair Implanter Carousel: a new surgical instrument for the automation of hair transplantation. Dermatol Surg 1998; 24:623-627.

10. Bernstein RM, Rassman WR. Dissecting microscope versus magnifying loupes with transillumination in the preparation of follicular unit grafts. A bilateral controlled study. Dermatol Surg 1998; 24:875-880.

11. Bernstein RM. A neighbor's view of the "follicular family unit." Hair Transplant Forum Intl 1998; 8(3):23-25.

12. Bernstein RM: Microscopophobia. Hair Transplant Forum Intl 1998; 8(5):23.

13. Bernstein RM, Rassman WR, Seager D, Shapiro R, et al. Standardizing the classification and description of follicular unit transplantation and mini-micrografting techniques. Dermatol Surg 1998; 24:957-963.

14. Bernstein RM: Blind graft production: value at what cost? Hair Transplant Forum Intl 1998; 8(6):28-29.

15. Bernstein RM, Rassman WR, Seager D, Unger WP, et al. The future in hair transplantation. J of Aesthetic Dermatol & Cosmetic Dermatol Surg 1999; 1(1):55-89.

16. Bernstein RM, Rassman WR. The logic of follicular unit transplantation. Dermatol Clinics 1999; 17 (2):277-295.

17. Bernstein RM. Unified terminology for hair transplantation. Hair Transplant Forum Intl 1999; 9(4):121-123.

18. Bernstein RM, Rassman WR. Hemostasis with minimal epinephrine. Hair Transplant Forum Intl 1999; 9(5):153.

19. Bernstein RM. A slot by any other name. Hair Transplant Forum Intl 1999; 9(6):175.

20. Bernstein RM, Rassman WR, Stough D. In support of follicular unit transplantation. Dermatol Surg 2000; 26(2):160-162.

21. Bernstein RM, Rassman WR. Limiting epinephrine in large hair transplant sessions. Hair Transplant Forum Intl 2000; 10(2):39-42.

22. Bernstein RM. What's in a name? Hair Transplant Forum Intl 2000; 10(2):59.

23. Bernstein RM, Rassman WR, Rashid N. A new suture for hair transplantation: Poliglecaprone 25. Dermatol Surg 2001; 27(1):5-11.

24. Bernstein RM, Rassman WR. Follicular unit graft yield using three different techniques. Hair Transplant Forum Intl 2001; 11(1):1,11-13.

25. Bernstein RM, Rassman WR, Rashid N, Shiell R, Ascione S. The art of repair. (Completed for Publication)

# NHI

# Photo Album

The pictures in this album are unretouched photos of patients treated by Physicians at the New Hair Institute. While photographs can be useful in illustrating the results that may be achieved with hair transplantation, photographs should not serve as your only reference when evaluating hair restoration procedures. We encourage you to attend NHI Open Houses and Seminars where you will be able to meet some of our former patients in person to help you decide if hair restoration surgery is right for you.

**All patients at the New Hair Institute are treated exclusively with Follicular Unit Transplantation.**

**You may find additional photos on our website:**

## newhair.com

# PATIENT FC

**Before and after
5,147 grafts**

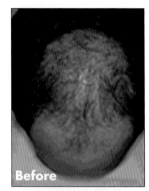

Before

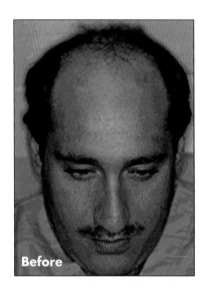

Before

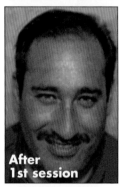

After
1st session

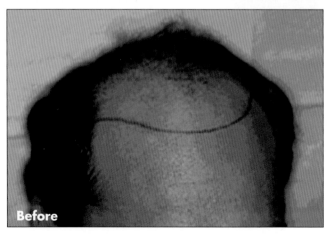

Before

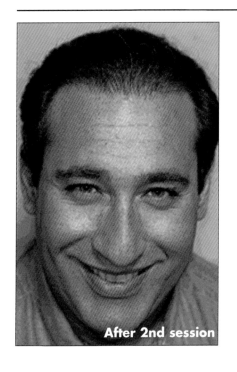

**After 2nd session**

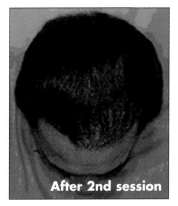

**After 2nd session**

Patient FC has dark brown hair. He was a Norwood Class 6 and had 2,747 grafts in the first session. He has a hair density of 2.8 hairs/mm$^2$ and was able to get excellent coverage. Note the soft, faded leading edge of the hairline. A second procedure of 2,400 follicular units was used to add density.

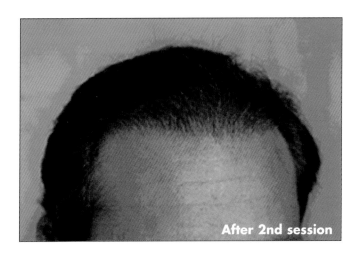

**After 2nd session**

Patient LF is a 48 year old male with an early Norwood Class 5A/6 pattern of hair loss. Existing hair in frontal region added to the fullness of the transplant. A dramatic change in his appearance was achieved after just one session of Follicular Unit Transplantation.

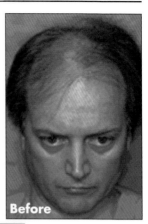

Before

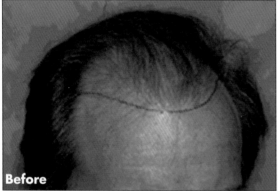

Before

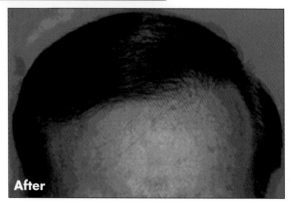

After

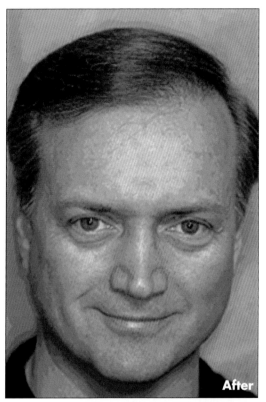

## PATIENT LF

**Before and after
one session of
2,803 grafts**

After

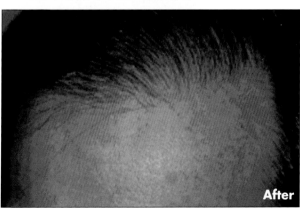

After

# PATIENT CF

## Before and after
## 3,686 grafts

Patient CF, a 38 year old, is a Norwood Class 5a/6 patient who received 3,686 grafts. His light blond hair and fair skin made him an excellent candidate for hair transplantation.

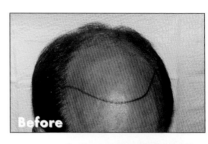

Before

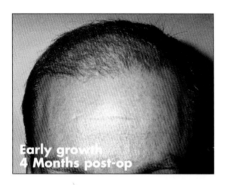

Early growth
4 Months post-op

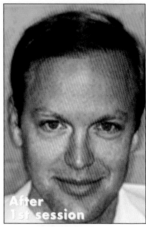

After
1st session

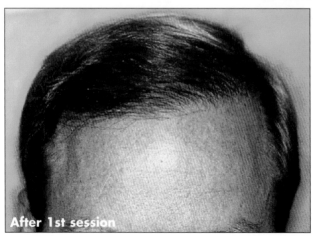

After 1st session

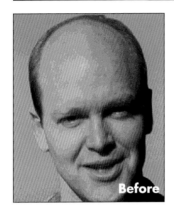

Before

Our patient was kind enough to allow us to use his photos for our article "The Aesthetics of Follicular Transplantation." As you can see, his results are incredible.

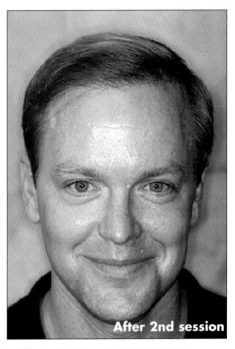

After 2nd session

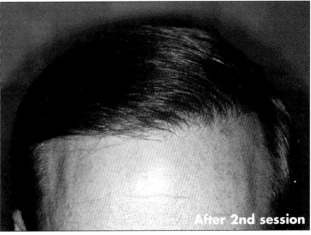

After 2nd session

# PATIENT NI
## Before and after 4,016 grafts

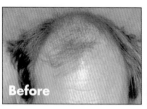

Before

NI is an Early Norwood Class 6 with medium-fine, light brown hair and a donor density of 2.1 hairs/mm². Photos were taken after two sessions of Follicular Unit Transplantation using 2,760 in the first session and 1,256 grafts in the second.

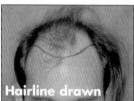

Hairline drawn

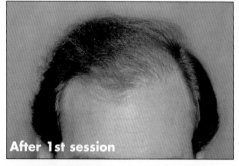

After 1st session

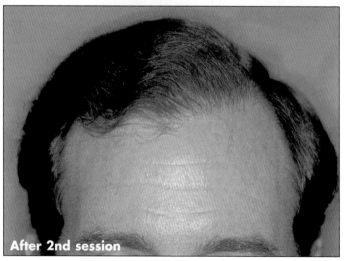

After 2nd session

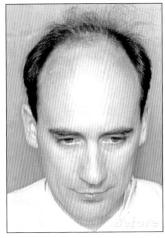

## PATIENT EC

**Before and after
one session of
1,750 grafts**

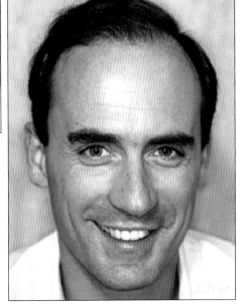

EC is a Norwood Class 5A-6 with brown, straight hair. Patient EC had old plugs on the top of his scalp, slightly visible in the before view and camouflaged with one session of Follicular Unit Transplantation using 1,750 grafts.

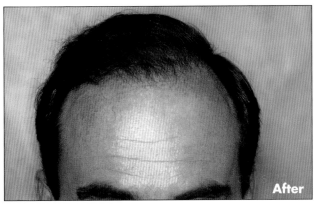

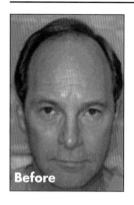

Before

Patient CC is a 51 year old dentist who had very definite ideas regarding how his hairline should be planned. His specific concern was that his temples would show enough recession for his age. Note how balanced and natural his final result looks. Photos taken one year after his second procedure showing younger appearance even now that he is older and wearing glasses.

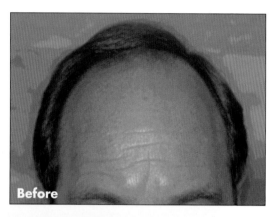

Before

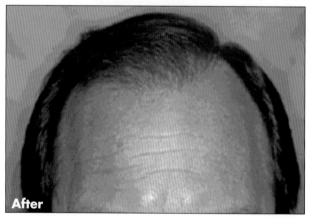

After

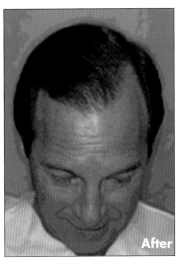

**After**

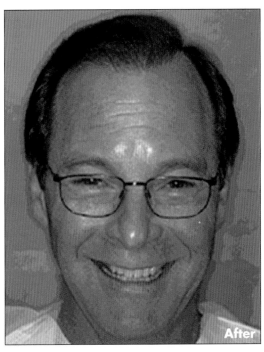

**After**

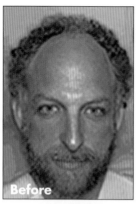

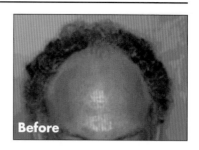

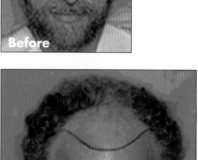

Mr. LK is a middle aged male with total frontal hair loss in a Norwood Class 4A pattern with enough thinning so that he is actually an early Class 6. He has curly brown hair of medium weight and slightly above average donor density. Results below are 15 months after one session of Follicular Unit Transplantation.

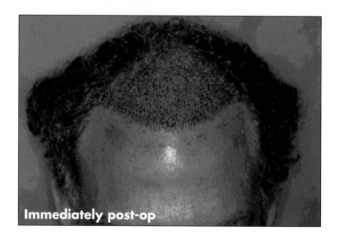

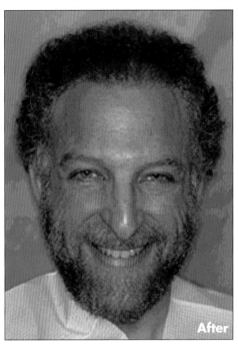

## PATIENT LK

**Before and after
one session of
2,228 grafts**

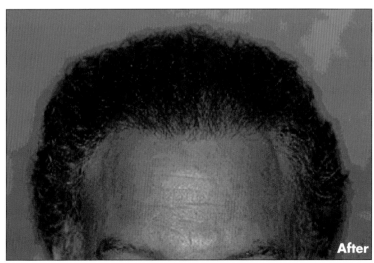

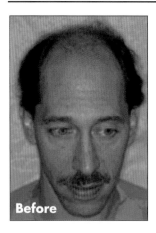

**Before**

# PATIENT LL

**Before and after
one session of
2,365 grafts**

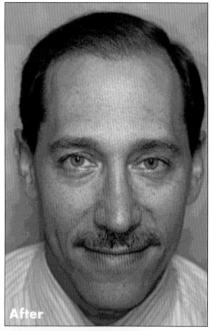

**After**

Mr. LL is in his early 40's with a norwood class 6 hair loss pattern. He has an average donor density. The results shown are 11 months after just one session of Follicular Unit Transplantation.

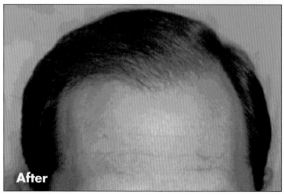

**After**

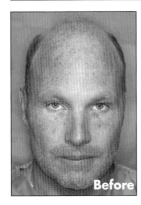
Before

EJ is a Norwood Class 6 with very fine, blonde hair and a donor density of 2.5 hairs/mm². He had two sessions of Follicular Unit Transplantation. A wave appeared after his second transplant – he hadn't had one for over twenty years.

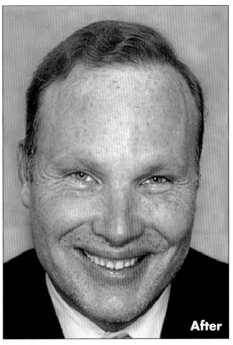
After

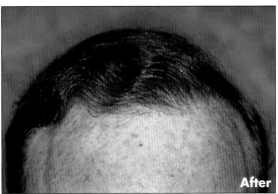
After

213

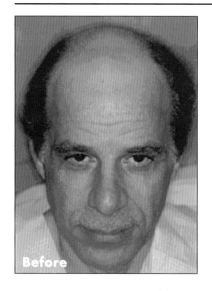
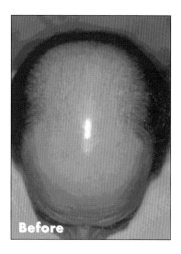

Mr. CK, a 54 year old Norwood Class 6/7, wore a toupee for many years. He has salt and pepper, slightly wavy, fine hair and an average donor density (2.0 hair/mm²). His first session consisted of 2,199 follicular units and a second session was used to increase density with an additional 1,459 follicular units.

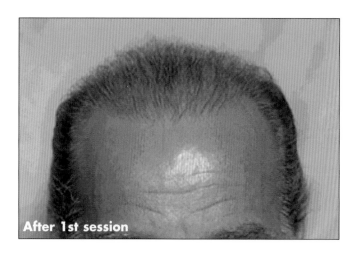

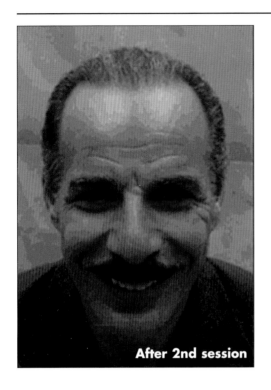

**PATIENT CK**
Before and after
3,658 grafts

After 2nd session

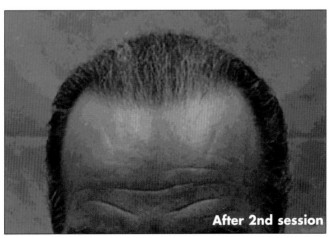

After 2nd session

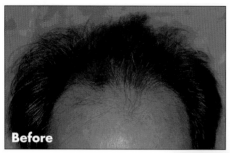

Before

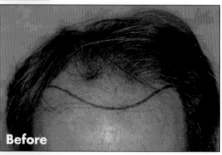

Before

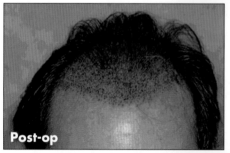

Post-op

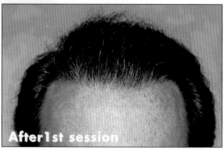

After 1st session

# PATIENT QS

## Before and after
## 3,523 grafts

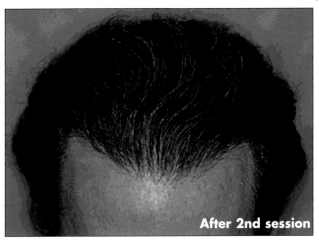

Mr. QS was a middle aged male with great hair characteristics and balding limited to the front part of his scalp
(Norwood 4A). Results shown are after one and two sessions of Follicular Unit Transplantation.

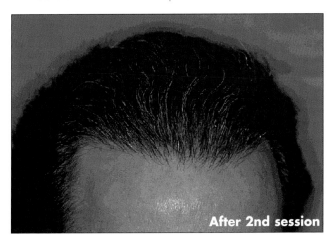

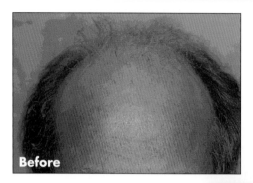

Before

Patient AQ is in his early 50's with medium weight, wiry, light brown hair with advanced Norwood Class 6 hair loss. Results shown are after 3 sessions of Follicular Unit Transplantation.

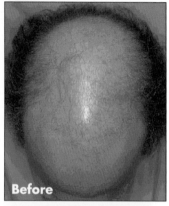

Before

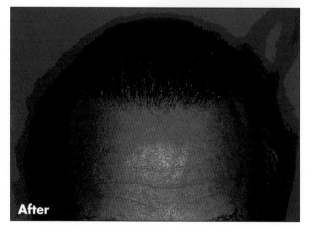

After

**Before and after
5,966 grafts**

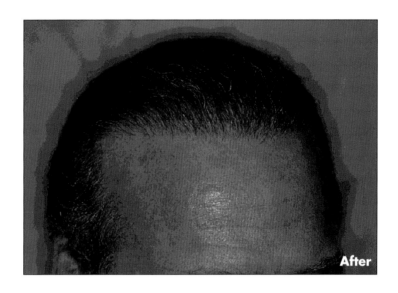

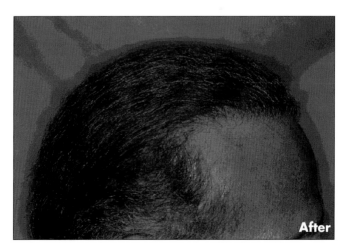

## PATIENT GI

**Before and after one session of 1,295 grafts**

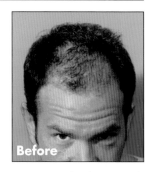

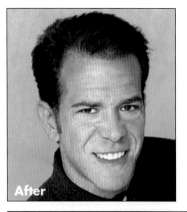

Patient GI was a Norwood Class 4 with brown, wavy hair of medium high density. Before his procedure, he always wore a baseball cap wherever he went. He now reports that all 20 of his caps are in storage. His friends told him he looks younger and asked if he had lost weight. Nobody detected his transplant... not even his hair stylist!

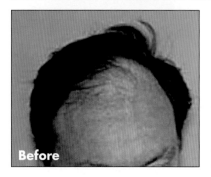

## PATIENT QQ

**Before and after one session of 2,025 grafts**

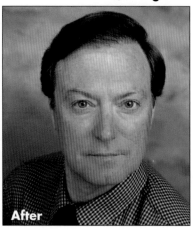

"The photos clearly showed that my comb-over was not working. After I had the one transplant procedure of 2,025 grafts, I looked at my before picture and I was shocked to see how bald I had really become. I never regretted for a moment what I had done. I just can't believe it took me so long to do it."

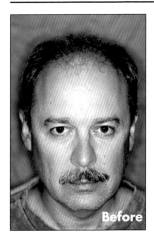
Before

## PATIENT ML
### Before and after one session of 2,520 grafts

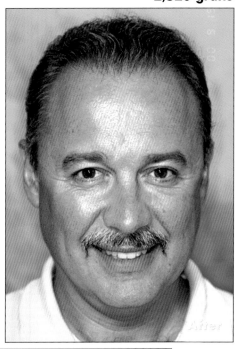

ML is an early Norwood class 6 with medium weight, wavy, salt & pepper hair. Photos taken after one session of follicular unit transplantation. A second session is planned to increase his density.

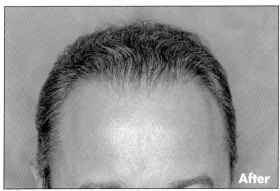
After

## PATIENT OD

### Before and after one session of 1,375 grafts

Patient OD was a Norwood Class 6 with a very sparse hairline. Notice that his appearance now reflects the full and natural hairline of a mature gentleman.

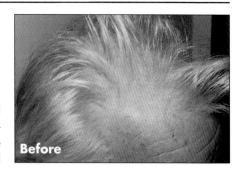

Before

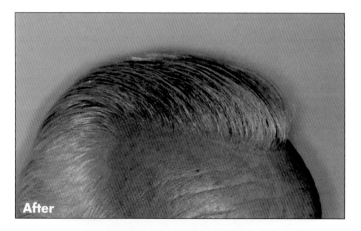

After

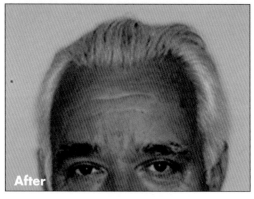

After

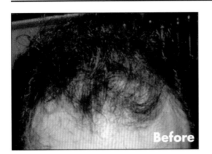

## PATIENT BZ
### Before and after one session of 1,440 grafts

Patient BZ was a Norwood Class 6 with black, curly hair. Most of the immediate loss focus was in the frontal area. This curly hair type covers the balding area very well and usually requires a lesser number of grafts.

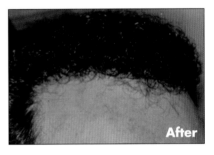

## PATIENT WR
### Before and after One session of 762 grafts

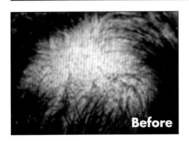

Dr. Rassman before and two years after 762 grafts.

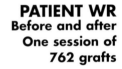

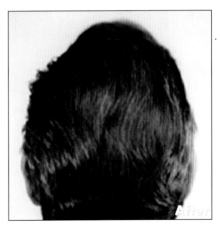

# PATIENT RF

**Before and after
2,712 grafts**

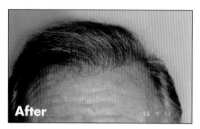

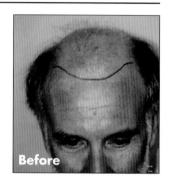

Patient RF was a Norwood Class 7 patient. He has gray hair and light skin. This is one of least difficult combinations for hair transplantation.  RF is very happy with his results.

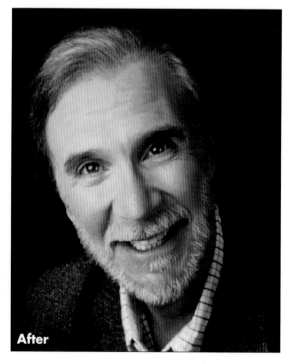

Mr. ID was Norwood Class 7 patient in his thirties. He had two sessions with a total of 4,040 grafts. The transplants were never detected and he was often complimented on his new hair styling.

## PATIENT ID
### Before and after 4,040 grafts

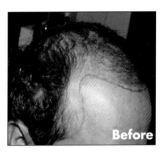

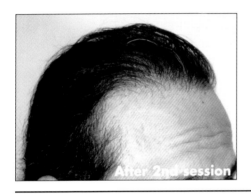

## PATIENT VV

### Before and after 4,240 grafts

Patient VV has dark brown hair and light fair skin with average hair density. He had three sessions over five years with a total of 4,240 follicular units transplanted.

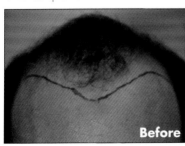

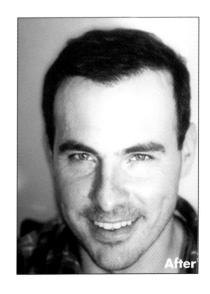

# PATIENT JF

**Before and after
3,116 grafts**

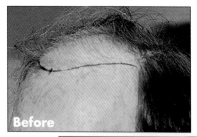

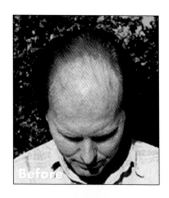

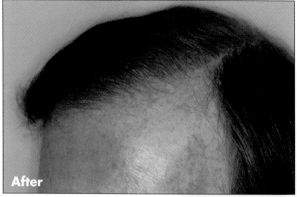

Mr. JF, an agriculturist, was a Norwood Class 5A patient. He has red hair and fair skin, and his results are excellent.

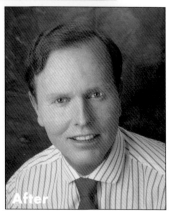

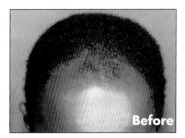

## PATIENT IQ
### Before and after
### 1,524 grafts

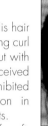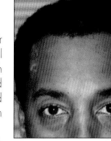

Mr. IQ was a Norwood Class 4A patient. His hair is typical of African American hair with a strong curl to it. His density was lower than average, but with his dark skin, the results are good. He received 1,524 grafts in two sessions. The patient exhibited no cobblestoning, a common complication in African Americans who have had large grafts.

"Baldness affected my motivation and self-confidence. I wore caps as often as possible in order to hide my receding hair line. I have had two procedures and my confidence and hair seemed to come back at about the same time."

## PATIENT LA
### Before and after
### 1,500 grafts

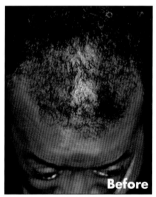

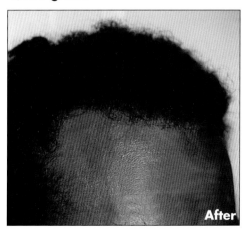

"I am very grateful. I accomplished the results shown above in two surgeries totaling 1,500 grafts."

227

# PATIENT RI

## Before and after
## 3,344 grafts

Patient RI was a Norwood Class 4 patient who received a total of 3,344 grafts in two sessions. He has brown hair and fair skin, and his results are excellent.

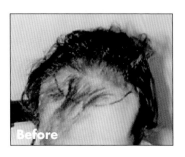

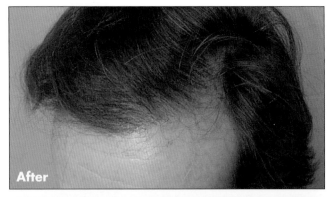

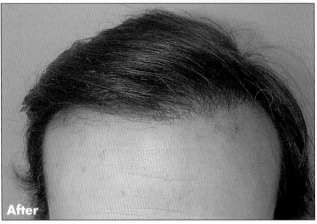

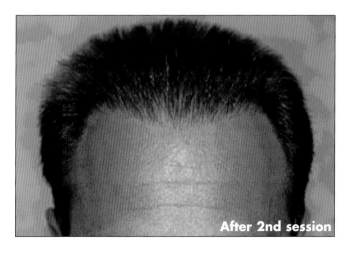

## PATIENT BL
### Before and after
### 4,559 grafts

Before

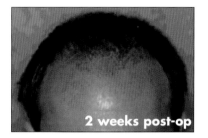

2 weeks post-op

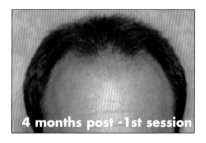

4 months post -1st session

(1) Above: Patient BL is in his late 30's with fine, brown hair, average scalp laxity, and a donor density of 2.5/mm². 
(2) Right (Upper): Two weeks after 1st session showing only the faint stubble of transplanted hair.
(3) Right (Lower): Very early growth after 1st session.
(4) Below: Result after 2nd session. A total of 4,559 grafts were transplanted in the two sessions.

After 2nd session

## PATIENT CQ
**Before and after
one session of
2,064 grafts**

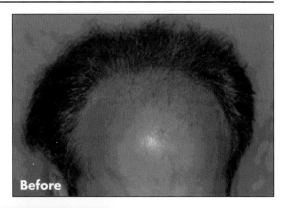

Before

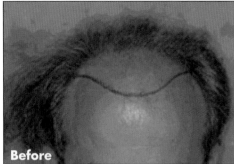

Before

Patient CQ has medium
weight, slightly wiry, brown,
salt and pepper hair.
Restoration was completed
in one session of 2,064 follicular units.

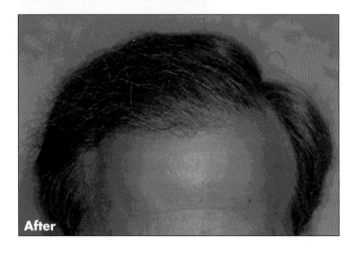

After

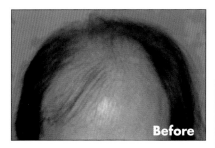

Before

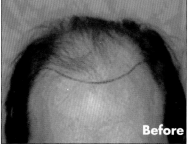

Before

Patient GF has very fine hair and shows good results after one procedure of 2,567 follicular units and great results after a second session of an additional 934 follicular units.

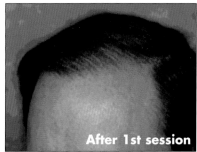

After 1st session

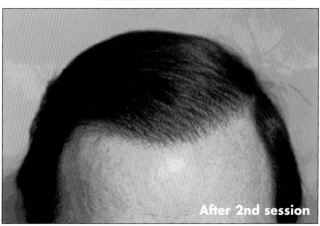

After 2nd session

# PATIENT LU

## Before and after one session of 928 grafts

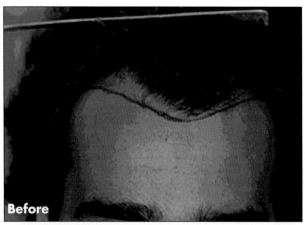

Before

Patient LU is in his mid 30's, with progression from an adolescent to a mature hairline that was bothered by the recession in the corners (Bi-temporal area). It is important to note that this type of restoration is only appropriate for patients with little risk of significant hair loss and an abundant donor supply.

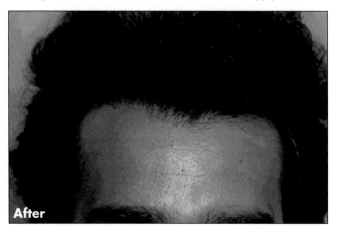

After

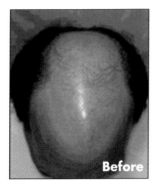

**Before**

## PATIENT JD
### Before and after one session of 2,292 grafts

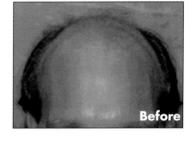

**Before**

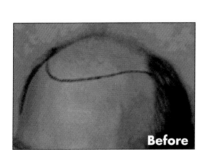

**Before**

Patient JD is in his mid 40's, and has light brown hair in a Norwood class 6 balding pattern. He wore a hairpiece for many years. Great results are seen with one session of Follicular Unit Transplantation. His hairline can be thickened further if he chooses.

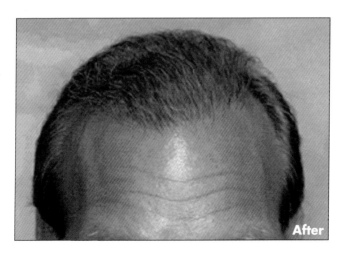

**After**

# PATIENT VS

**Before and after
1,656 grafts**

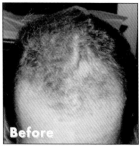

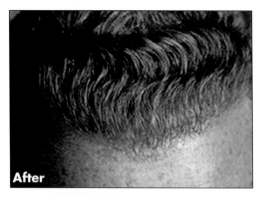

Patient VS was a Norwood Class 4A patient with dark blonde hair. Note that the hairline is not a line, but a zone reflecting a gradation of hair from the forehead to the thicker hair behind.

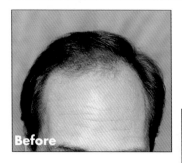

# PATIENT GR

**Before and after
3,087 grafts**

GR was a Norwood Class 4 with very fine, light brown, straight hair and a donor density of 2.8 hairs/mm$^2$. "After" photo was taken after two sessions of follicular unit transplantation using 1,241 and 1,846 grafts.

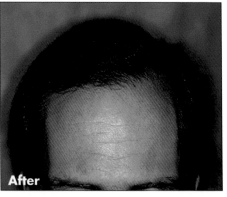

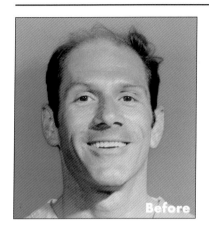

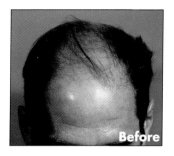

## PATIENT GO
**Before and after
3,688 grafts**

Patient GO was a Norwood Class 6 patient with wavy brown hair. When GO came to the office for a follow-up visit, no one recognized him!

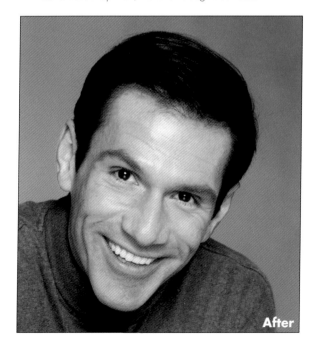

235

## PATIENT KI

### Before and after one session of 894 grafts

Patient KI was a Norwood Class 4A. The 'After' photos were taken 10 months after his second procedure. KI has a 'thin' frontal hairline which can be thickened further if he chooses.

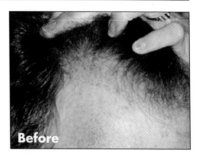

Before

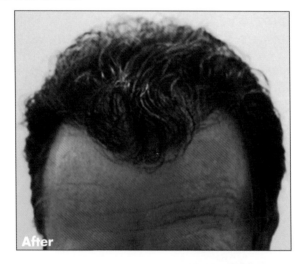

After

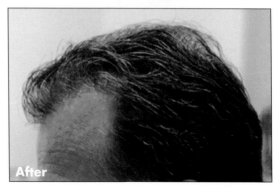

After

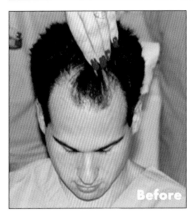

## PATIENT QK
### Before and after one session of 1,393 grafts

**Before**

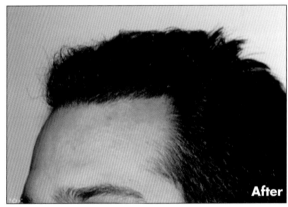

**After**

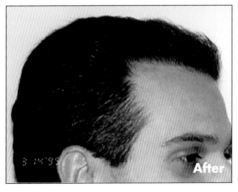

**After**

Patient QK was a Norwood Class 4A with black, coarse, straight hair. Some years before coming to NHI, he received 80 large plugs that, fortunately, never grew. This left him less pluggy than had they grown. NHI placed 1,393 grafts in one session. Notice the growth of the hair, the natural appearance and the distribution of the grafts.

# PATIENT EK

**Before and after
2,577 grafts**

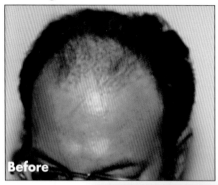

Mr. EK was a Norwood Class 5 with curly light brown hair. As you can see, his coverage is excellent. Prior to his procedure, he was wearing a hairpiece which did not fit into his lifestyle. Mr. EK was bald in front and bald in back. The two bald areas used to be separated by a one-inch bridge of hair.

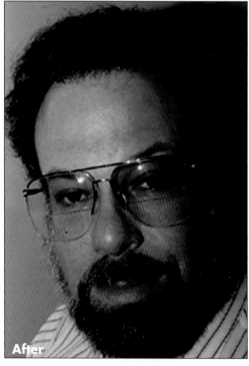

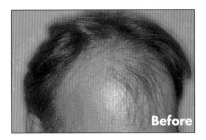

Before

## PATIENT IF

### Before and after one session of 1,810 grafts

Patient IF is in mid 40's with straight, light brown hair of medium weight with frontal hair loss, Norwood Class 4A. His donor density at 2.4 hairs/mm² is above average.

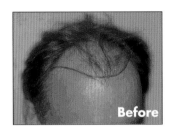

Before

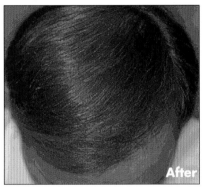

After

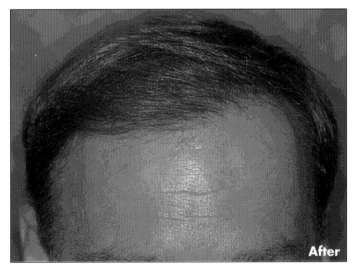

After

## PATIENT RM

**Before and after one session of 210 grafts**

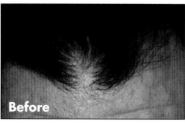

Before

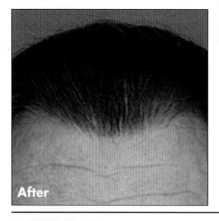

After

Dr. McClellan, a NHI surgeon, developed some thinning hair in front at 40. He had surgery at another clinic, but developed a bald spot in his forelock as well as further thinning on his left side. He had 100 grafts placed very closely together in the widow's peak and 110 grafts more widely scattered on the left side.

## PATIENT RF

**Before and after 2,880 grafts**

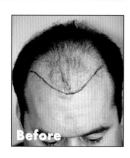

Before

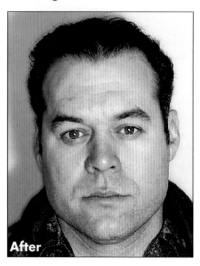

After

Patient RF was a Norwood Class 6 patient with dark brown hair. He received 2,880 grafts in two sessions and is very happy with his results. No one ever detected that he had a hair transplantation procedure.

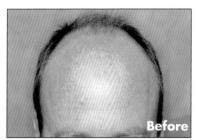

**Before**

# PATIENT JQ
## Before and after
## 3,324 grafts

JQ is a Norwood Class 6 with blond hair. Photos were taken after two sessions of follicular unit transplantation using 1,769 and 1,555 grafts.

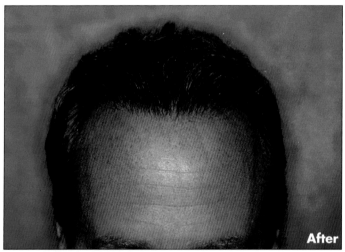

**After**

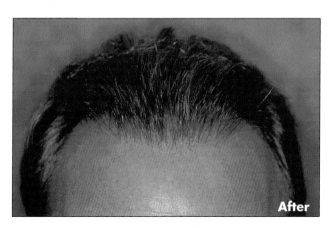

**After**

## PATIENT LB

**Before and after one session of 1,574 grafts**

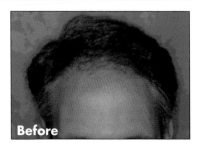

Before

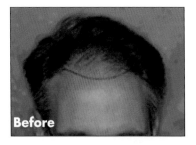

Before

Mr. LB is a 41 year old Norwood Class 3A/4A with good hair characteristics. Results after one session of Follicular Unit Transplantation. The 'Post-op' photo illustrates the gentleness of the procedure.

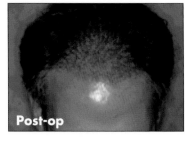

Post-op

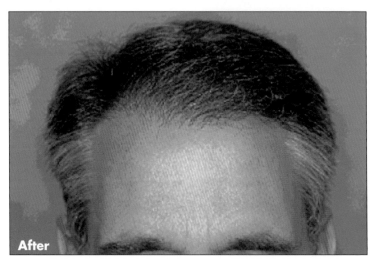

After

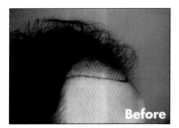

Before

## PATIENT GI
### Before and after
### 2,170 grafts

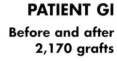

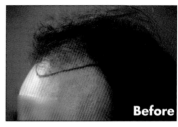

Before

"Dr. Rassman has terrific presence and is very concerned for people's well-being. I choose NHI because I thought that if he could transplant a heart successfully, he could handle my transplant!"

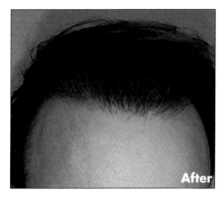

After

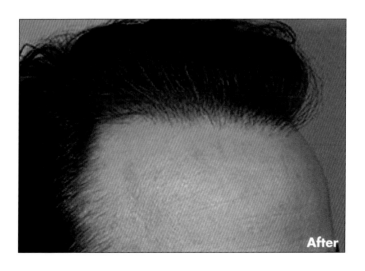

After

# PATIENT FI

## Before and after one session of 1,290 grafts

FI was a Norwood Class 4A with medium weight, straight brown hair. "After" photos taken after one session of follicular unit transplantation of 1,210 grafts. Larger "After photo shows mass of transplanted hair hanging forward.

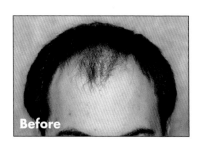

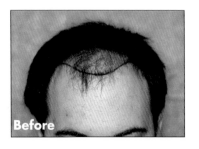

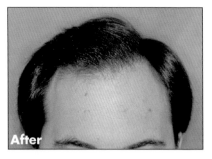

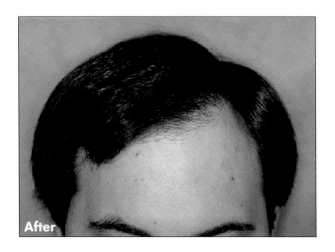

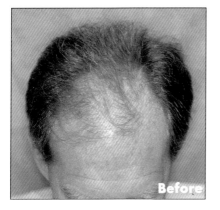

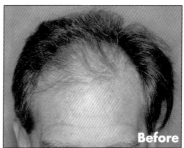

## PATIENT QA
### Before and after
### 2,963 grafts

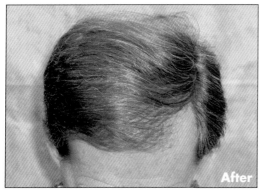

QA was a Norwood Class 5 with medium-fine, light brown hair. Photos taken after two sessions of follicular unit transplantation using 1,842 and 1,121 grafts.

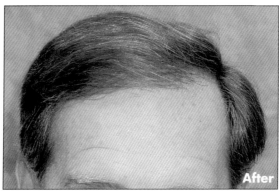

## PATIENT MA

### Before and after one session of 1,801 grafts

MA is a Norwood Class 5A with medium weight, wavy, salt & pepper hair. Photos were taken after one session of follicular unit transplantation. A second session was recently performed using an additional 1,450 grafts (not shown).

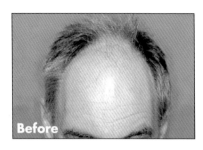

Before

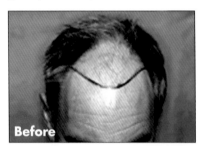

Before

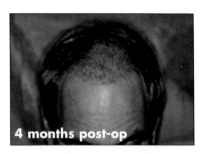

4 months post-op

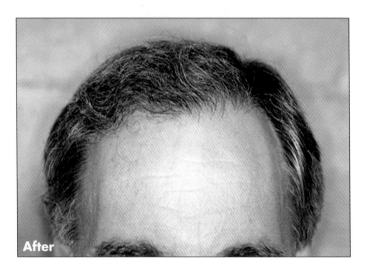

After

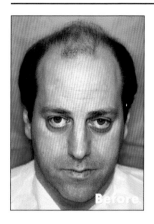

**Before and after
two sessions of
4,043 grafts**

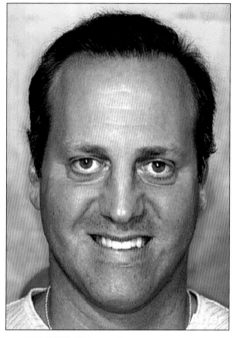

SU is an Early Norwood Class 6 with straight, brown hair. Photos taken after two sessions of Follicular Unit Transplantation using 2,377 and 1,666 grafts, spaced 15 months apart.

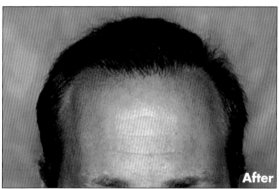

247

# PATIENT ES

**Before and after
3,030 grafts**

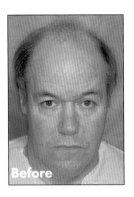

Before

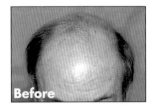

Before

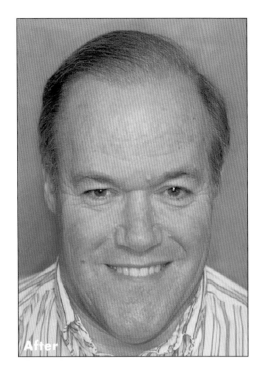

After

ES is a Norwood Class 6 with very fine, light brown hair and a donor density of 1.8 hairs/mm². He had two sessions of Follicular Unit Transplantation of 1,972 and 1,056 grafts that gave him light, but wonderfully natural coverage.

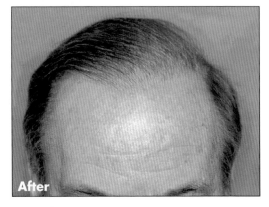

After

## PATIENT UQ

**Before and after
one session of
2,355 grafts**

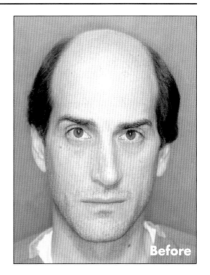

Before

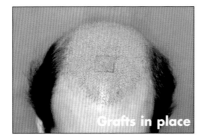

Grafts in place

UQ was a Norwood Class 6 with straight, medium-fine, dark brown hair of average density. The above photo shows grafts placed at an average of 20 follicular units/cm$^2$. The box shows the area where the largest follicular units were used. The "after" photo was taken after a single session of 2,355 follicular unit grafts. Note the dramatic change in appearance, and completely natural look, after just one session. A second, smaller session will be performed to increase the density, especially at the frontal hairline.

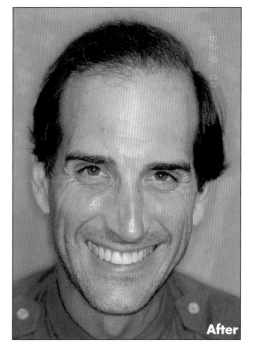

After

# PATIENT JQ

**Before and after one session of 1,491 grafts**

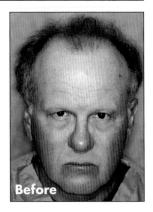

Before

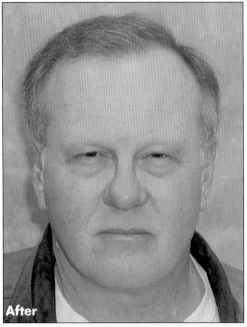

After

JQ is a Norwood Class 6 with medium weight slightly wiry hair and a donor density of 1.8 hairs/mm². These photos were taken after one session of Follicular Unit Transplantation.

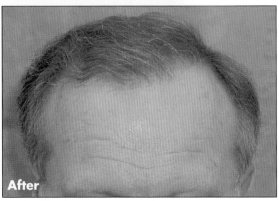

After

## PATIENT OE

**Before and after
1,800 grafts**

Patient OE is a Norwood cass 4. The after picture was taken 4 1/2 months after surgery, however results like this are usually seen in a timespan of six months.

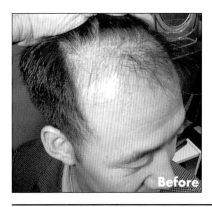

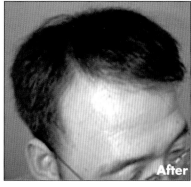

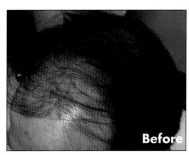

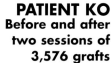

## PATIENT KO
**Before and after
two sessions of
3,576 grafts**

KO is a Norwood Class 6 with straight medium weight hair. These photos were taken after two sessions of Follicular Unit Transplantation

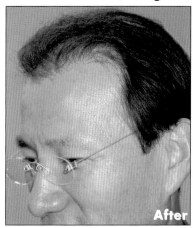

# REPAIRS

### These people are <u>now</u> NHI patients.

## PATIENT LE

### Graft excision and reimplantation: Step-by-step

(1) A row of plugs at the frontal hairline

(2) Plug removal using 2.5–3mm punches

(3) Sutured sites after the removal (note the hair re-transplanted to the front edge of the old hairline)

(4) Some residual white scars from the plugs

(5) Intra-operative view of the 1st transplant of 1,374, with grafts placed directly into the scarred area

(6) Results 11 months after 1st session

(7) Final result after 3 sessions

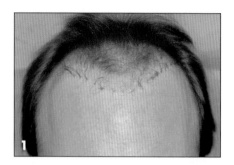

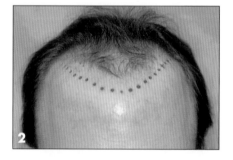

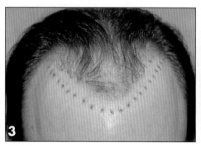

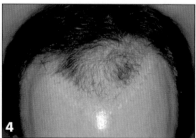

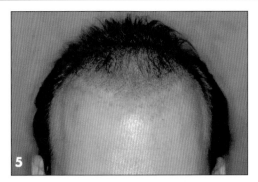

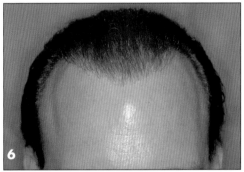

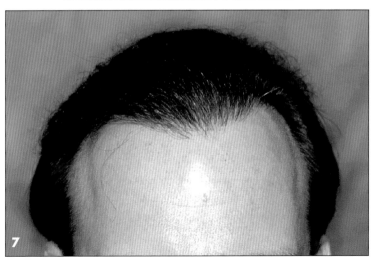

# REPAIRS

**These people are <u>now</u> NHI patients.**

## PATIENT RI

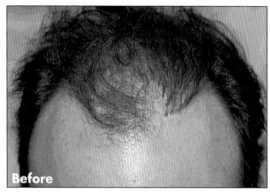

Before

Plugs placed within patients old hairline by another transplant center were not too noticeable at first. However, with further hair loss, the poorly planned transplant became very unnatural. Fortunately for the patient, the old plugs were located high enough so that a dramatic camouflage was achieved with just one session of Follicular Unit Transplantation.

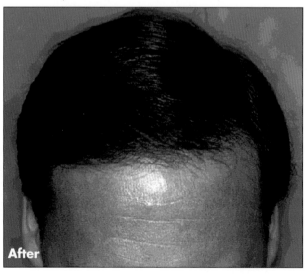

After

# REPAIRS

**These people are <u>now</u> NHI patients.**

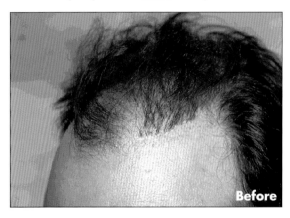

Before

These pictures were taken at the same time at a slightly different angle; illustrating the striking linearity of the original grafts.

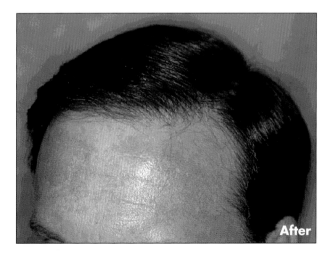

After

# REPAIRS

**These people are <u>now</u> NHI patients.**

## PATIENT BI

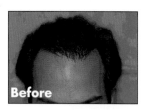
Before

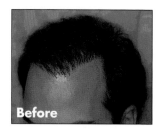
Before

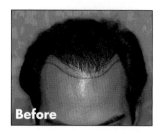
Before

Patient BI has medium weight hair of above average density (2.5/mm²). Two original sessions of large mini-grafts resulted in a hairline that was too lop-sided and pluggy. Patient was treated at NHI with two sessions of Follicular Unit Transplantation and some of the largest mini-grafts in the very front were removed. The hair from these grafts were subdivided under the microscope and re-implanted. We always use every single follicle!

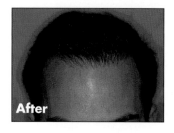
After

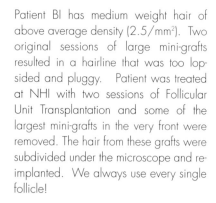
After

# REPAIRS

**These people are <u>now</u> NHI patients.**

## PATIENT CZ

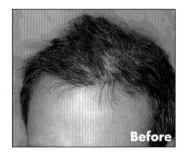

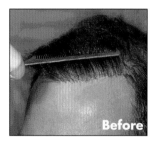

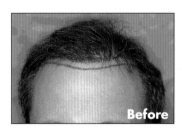

Patient CZ came to NHI for the repair of very uniform, unnatural frontal hairline. This was achieved with two sessions of Follicular Unit Transplantation.

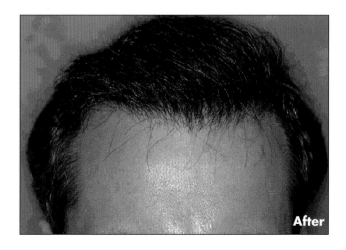

# REPAIRS

### These people are <u>now</u> NHI patients.

## PATIENT ZO

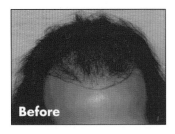

Mr. ZO originally had mini-grafts performed near his frontal hairline that became visible with further recession. Significant cosmetic improvement is seen with just one session of Follicular Unit Transplantation.

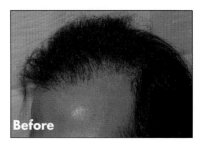

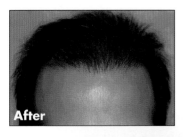

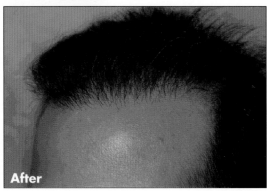

# REPAIRS

**These people are <u>now</u> NHI patients.**

## PATIENT JH

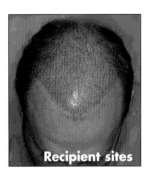

Recipient sites

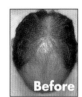

Before

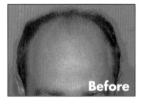

Before

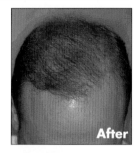

After

Four Y-shaped scalp reductions left a large geometric scar on the top of the head and a tightened scalp, which made future transplantation difficult. The top photo shows the distribution of recipient sites for the new grafts. The last two photos show the results after one session of 1,825 follicular units. A second procedure may be used to achieve greater density if he chooses.

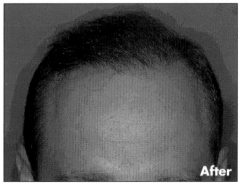

After

# REPAIRS

**These people are <u>now</u> NHI patients.**

## PATIENT KL

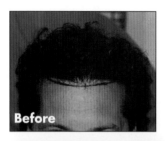

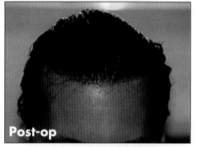

Mr. KL is a 33 year old male with a Class 3 hair pattern. He had undergone surgery 5 times in the past. He wanted to normalize the hairline and increase the density in the front. The first picture shows the planned hairline and the second shows the results immediately after the first surgery, when 1,010 grafts were placed. The third picture shows the results after a second procedure of 612 grafts and 3 years of growth.

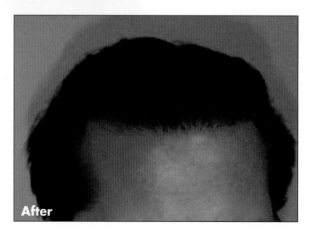

# REPAIRS

**These people are <u>now</u> NHI patients.**

## PATIENT SZ

Patient SZ came to NHI for repair work. Scars contract as they heal, so when larger grafts are placed into scalpel incisions as shown, the grafts squeeze together. The hairs which grow from these sites look like ferns growing in a forest as they appear to grow from a single hole. Patient SZ paid over $10,000 for his pluggy look. NHI placed 1,500 grafts to camouflage the problem.

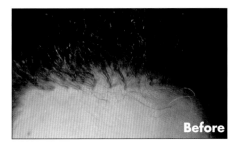

Before

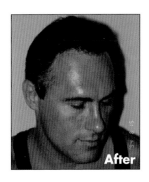

After

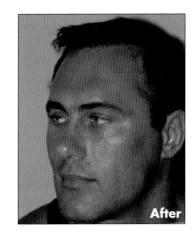

After

# REPAIRS

**These people are <u>now</u> NHI patients.**

## PATIENT QB

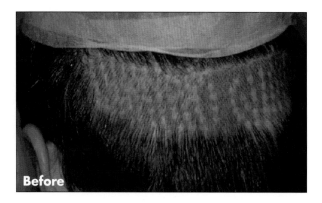

Grafts harvested from area of extensive scarring (from the old open donor technique) using the newer single strip method. Note how the area of scarring is dramatically reduced. The tissue removed will be placed under a dissecting microscope so that all of the viable hair follicles will be preserved.

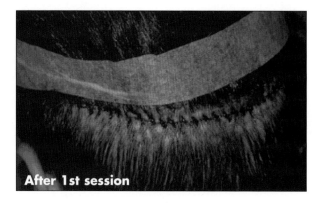

# REPAIRS

## These people are <u>now</u> NHI patients.

## PATIENT OI

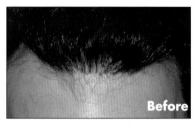

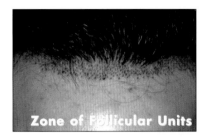

Three sessions of Follicular Unit Transplantation were used to soften this person's harsh frontal hairline.

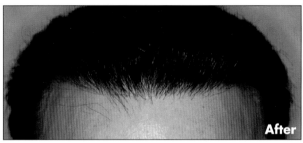

---

## PATIENT KQ

"Previous 'plug' procedure by another company left me looking weird. NHI performed 1,016 grafts and now I am normal again."

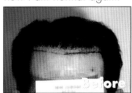

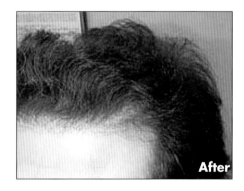

# REPAIRS

**These people are <u>now</u> NHI patients.**

## PATIENT AQ

Mr. AQ had old plugs that failed to grow hair. Note the visible white scars produced by the hairless plugs. After the repair with one procedure of Follicular Unit Transplantation, the scarring was undetectable and the patient let his hair grow naturally gray.

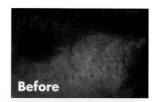

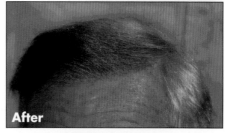

## PATIENT AS

Mr. AS had a very pluggy frontal hairline from the old plug technique. A slight Widow's Peak was created to break up the straight-line appearance of the hairline and to camouflage the plugs. This repair was accomplished with just one session of Follicular Unit Transplantation.

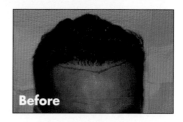

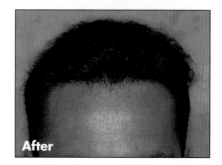

# REPAIRS
### These people are <u>now</u> NHI patients.

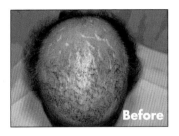

## PATIENT JG

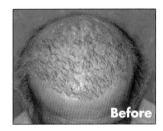

Patient JG had extensive scarring from a sew-on hairpiece and 3 hair transplant sessions using plugs, many of which didn't grow well. Luckily, the patient had salt & pepper hair, ideal hair for a repair. Dramatic improvement was accomplished with just one session, although a second session is planned. One problem that we could not correct was the very low hairline.

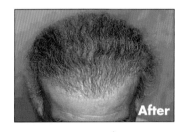

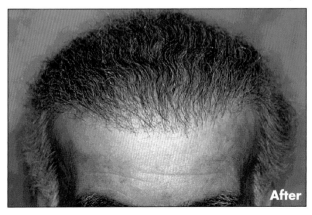

# REPAIRS

**These people are <u>now</u> NHI patients.**

## PATIENT QI

Three sessions of Follicular Unit Transplantation were used to soften this person's dense row of plugs.

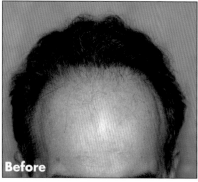

Before

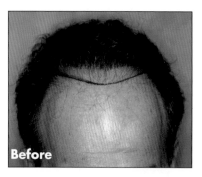

Before

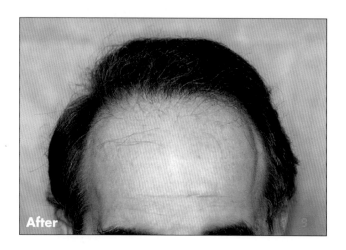

After

# WHAT TO AVOID
## These were <u>NOT</u> NHI patients.

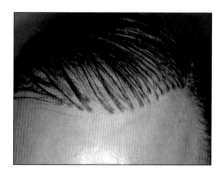

### DOLL'S HEAD APPEARANCE
This man is a "living doll." His unacceptable result of being plugged is worse than baldness, it is a travesty!

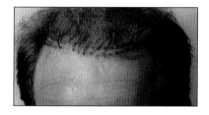

### DOLL'S HEAD APPEARANCE
This patient underwent a procedure of 40 grafts in the hairline with another center. This is the look you get when you "just get a few to see how you like them."

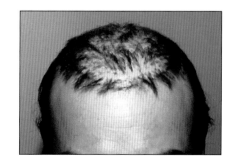

### DOLL'S HEAD APPEARANCE

# WHAT TO AVOID

**These were <u>NOT</u> NHI patients.**

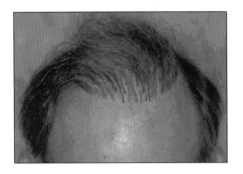

**DOLL'S HEAD APPEARANCE**

**DOLL'S HEAD APPEARANCE**
Very pluggy frontal hairline. The frontal view (shown above) is a common problem of the old plug technique. The inefficient use of the patient's donor supply leaves much of the scalp unfinished (at right).

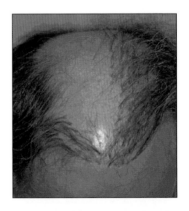

**DOLL'S HEAD APPEARANCE**
Although the patient was never happy with the plugs, his appearance dramatically worsened as his hairline receded.

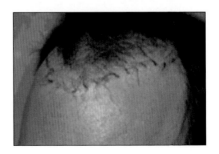

# WHAT TO AVOID
## These were **NOT** NHI patients.

### COBBLESTONING

This deformity of the skin is seen in larger grafts and remains visible until the hair grows in. It is present in virtually 100% of patients having larger grafts. If the hair does not cover the defects, the deformity is quite visible in bright light.

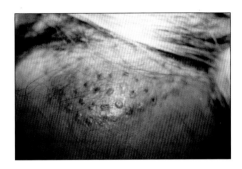

### COBBLESTONING

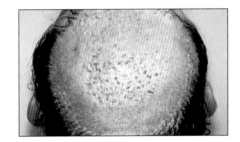

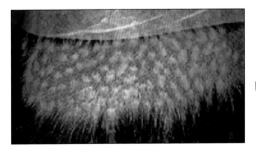

### EXTENSIVE SCARRING

Extensive open donor scarring.

# WHAT TO AVOID
## These were **NOT** NHI patients.

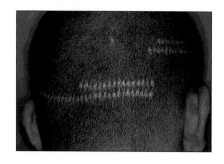

### EXTENSIVE SCARRING
Open donor scarring making it difficult for the patient to wear his hair short.

### SCALP REDUCTION
Midline scalp reduction with scarring and problems of altered hair direction.

### SCALP REDUCTION
Midline scalp reduction with an unusually deep indentation at the point of closure.

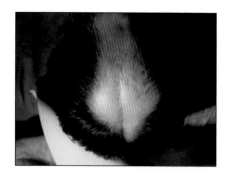

# WHAT TO AVOID
### These were <u>NOT</u> NHI patients.

**SCALP REDUCTION**

Complications of a poorly planned scalp reduction, that produced a wide scar and a 'Dog Ear' puckering of the scalp.

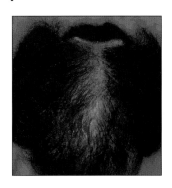

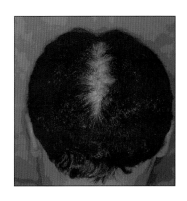

**SCALP REDUCTION**

Mercedes–Type Scarring from a scalp reduction.

**SCALP REDUCTION**

Scalp reduction producing a 'hatchet-like' scar in the back of the head.

# About the Authors

## William R. Rassman, M.D.

Dr. William R. Rassman graduated from the Medical College of Virginia in 1966 where he received his Doctor of Medicine. He completed a surgical internship at the University of Minnesota and proceeded with a cardiovascular fellowship with Dr. C.W. Lillehei. Dr. Rassman completed his residency in general surgery at Cornell Medical Center and Dartmouth Medical Center. He served as a surgeon in the U.S. Army during the Vietnam Conflict, attained the rank of Major, and was awarded a Silver Star. Dr. Rassman was certified by the American Board of Surgery in 1976.

Dr. Rassman was a major researcher in the cardiac field, and his work resulted in the commercialization of the Intra-Aortic Balloon Pump in 1969 that continues to save thousands of lives each year. He has authored many published articles and has written chapters in two textbooks in the cardiac field. As an inventor with both U.S. and international patents, Dr Rassman invented the Densitometer™ used in hair restoration for the precise measurement of hair density and hair quality. He also developed the Fast Track® method for hair transplantation where the hair restoration process can be completed, often in just one or two sessions. He holds multiple patents in computer software, the medical device industry, and in the hair transplantation field.

Dr. Rassman is motivated to make a difference. He strives for the best and is never satisfied with the status quo. He is a visionary and has never limited what he can accomplish by what has been done before. In the hair transplant field he has pioneered new techniques, published on them in peer

272